This book is dedicated to the fruitage of
25 years of teaching—my students.

# *The* EXERCISE- HEALTH CONNECTION

## David C. Nieman, DrPH

Appalachian State University

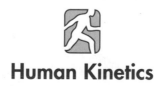

## Human Kinetics

**Library of Congress Cataloging-in-Publication Data**

Nieman, David C., 1950-
    The exercise health connection / David C. Nieman.
        p.    cm.
    Includes bibliographical references and index.
    ISBN 0-88011-584-X
    1. Exercise--Popular works.    2. Exercise therapy--Popular works.
    3. Health.    I. Title.
    RA781.N54    1997
    613.7'1--dc21                                                        97-36227
                                                                            CIP

ISBN:  0-88011-584-X

**Developmental Editors:** Holly Gilly and Kent Reel; **Assistant Editor:** Rebecca Crist; **Editorial Assistant:** Laura Ward Majersky; **Copyeditor:** Joyce Sexton; **Proofreader:** Sarah Wiseman; **Indexer:** Prottsman Indexing; **Graphic Designer:** Robert Reuther; **Graphic Artist:** Denise Lowry; **Cover Designer:** Stuart Cartwright; **Illustrator:** Tim Shedelbower; **Printer:** Versa Press

Human Kinetics books are available at special discounts for bulk purchase. Special editions or book excerpts can also be created to specification. For details, contact the Special Sales Manager at Human Kinetics.

Printed in the United States of America        10   9   8   7   6   5   4   3   2   1

**Human Kinetics**
Web site: http://www.humankinetics.com/

*United States:* Human Kinetics, P.O. Box 5076, Champaign, IL 61825-5076
1-800-747-4457
e-mail: humank@hkusa.com

*Canada:* Human Kinetics, Box 24040, Windsor, ON  N8Y 4Y9
1-800-465-7301 (in Canada only)
e-mail: humank@hkcanada.com

*Europe:* Human Kinetics, P.O. Box IW14, Leeds LS16 6TR, United Kingdom
(44) 1132 781708
e-mail: humank@hkeurope.com

*Australia:* Human Kinetics, 57A Price Avenue, Lower Mitcham, South Australia 5062
(088) 277 1555
e-mail: humank@hkaustralia.com

*New Zealand:* Human Kinetics, P.O. Box 105-231, Auckland 1
(09) 523 3462
e-mail: humank@hknewz.com

# CONTENTS

## Chapter 18   **Stress Management**                              **245**

## PART III   PHYSICAL ACTIVITY AND THE LIFE CYCLE                 263

## Chapter 19   **Children and Youth**                             **265**

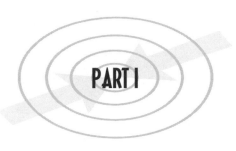

# PART I

# Physical Activity, Health, and the Human Body

In part I, a description of what it means to be healthy and physically fit will be given. Also, the major effects of exercise training on the human body will be outlined, with consideration given to the influence of genetics, gender, and age.

# Chapter 1

# PHYSICAL ACTIVITY COMPONENTS AND HEALTH

The "positiveness" of health does not lie in the state,
but in the struggle—the effort to reach a goal
which in its perfection is unattainable.

*Lancet* 2 (1958): 638

If I told you that I had a formula that would help you live longer, avoid—and even cure—some diseases, relieve stress, and make you stronger with virtually no bad side effects, you'd probably be willing to pay a lot of money for it. But what if I told you it was free? You'd probably be a little skeptical and say to yourself "It's too good to be true," "Nobody gets something for nothing," or "If it's that great, why doesn't everybody have it?"

The truth is, I do have a formula like that, and it doesn't cost any money. But you can't get it for nothing. You have to make an investment. The formula is physical activity—simple exercise. And, if you invest at least 30 minutes three times a week in moderately vigorous activity, you *can* get the benefits I described.

So the question still remains, "If it's that great, why doesn't everybody have it?" You're probably aware, from your own experiences and from looking at the people you're in contact with, that most Americans aren't making that investment. Fewer than 4 in 10 Americans exercise enough to get those health benefits. The purpose of this book is to show you the evidence from scientific research proving that regular physical activity lowers the risk for many diseases, strengthens most body systems, and improves psychological health. When you see the evidence, I hope you'll be willing to make the investment.

## HEALTH AND FITNESS DEFINED

Health is defined as a state of complete physical, mental, social, and spiritual well-being, and not merely the absence of disease and infirmity. Physical fitness is a condition in which an individual has sufficient energy and vitality to accomplish daily tasks and active recreational pursuits without undue fatigue.

The end objective in promoting physical activity is health. The most notable, and undoubtedly still the most influential, definition of health is that of the World Health Organization (WHO). The definition appeared in the preamble of the WHO constitution during the late 1940s: "Health is a state of complete physical, mental, and social well-being, and not merely the absence of disease and infirmity."

Figure 1.1 presents the concept of the "Health Continuum." Each individual can position him- or herself somewhere on this passage between health and death. On the left side of the continuum is health as defined by WHO. The absence of health is death, as depicted on the right side. For most people, before death comes disease, which itself is preceded by a sustained period of high-risk behaviors. Health represents a dynamic state of positive well-being in which one follows habits that promote health, lowering the risk of premature disease and death.

Physical health and fitness is a positive quality that is related to the prevention of most of the diseases listed in figure 1.1. Physical fitness places an emphasis on having vigor and energy to perform physical work and exercise. Physical fitness can be subjectively measured by determining how much energy one has for doing what is enjoyable in life and for experiencing all the natural adventure possible. Engaging in activities from snow skiing to mountain climbing, cycling to weekend backpacking, those who are physically fit have the energy and zest to maximize their enjoyment of the natural resources available to them.

Vigor and energy are not easily measured, however, and experts have debated for more than a century the important measurable components of physical fitness. As will be emphasized in the next section, when people exercise regularly in such a way as to keep their heart, lungs, and skeletal muscles in shape while keeping lean, most authorities would equate this with physical fitness.

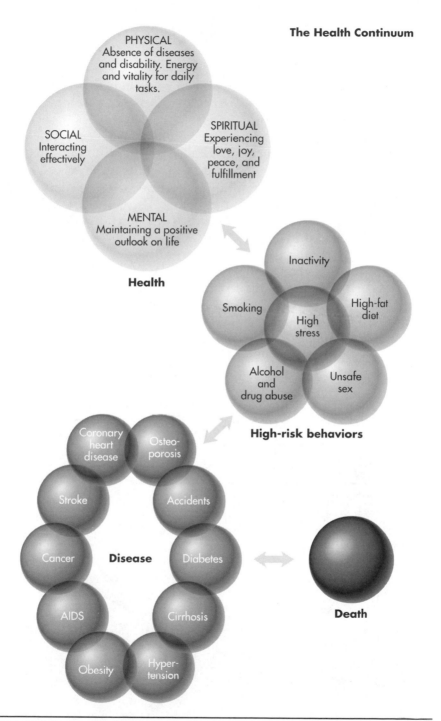

**The Health Continuum**

PHYSICAL
Absence of diseases
and disability. Energy
and vitality for daily
tasks.

SPIRITUAL
Experiencing
love, joy,
peace, and
fulfillment

SOCIAL
Interacting
effectively

MENTAL
Maintaining a positive
outlook on life

**Health**

Inactivity

Smoking

High
stress

High-fat
diet

Alcohol
and
drug abuse

Unsafe
sex

**High-risk behaviors**

Coronary
heart
disease

Osteo-
porosis

Stroke

Accidents

Cancer

**Disease**

Diabetes

AIDS

Cirrhosis

Obesity

Hyper-
tension

**Death**

FIGURE 1.1 For most people, before death comes disease, which itself is preceded by a sustained period of high-risk behaviors.

# COMPONENTS OF HEALTH-RELATED FITNESS

Health-related physical fitness is typified by an ability to perform daily activities with vigor and is related to a low risk of chronic disease. Cardiorespiratory endurance, musculoskeletal fitness (muscular strength and endurance, flexibility), and optimal body composition are the measurable components of health-related fitness. Skill-related fitness, on the other hand, has more to do with agility, balance, coordination, speed, power, and reaction time (sport skills) and has little relationship to health and disease prevention.

The most frequently cited components of physical fitness fall into two groups, one related to health and the other related to athletic skills (see figure 1.2). Skill-related fitness is integral to success in sports such as tennis, football, baseball, volleyball, golf, and basketball. However, most experts feel that these components have little if any bearing on health and disease prevention. For example, there are no scientific data to suggest that coordinated people live longer or suffer less disease than uncoordinated people.

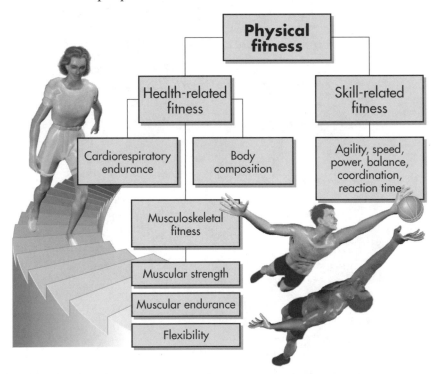

FIGURE 1.2    Physical fitness has both health- and skill-related components.

Health-related fitness includes these components:

- **Cardiorespiratory fitness:** the ability to continue or persist in strenuous tasks involving large muscle groups for extended periods of time. Also called aerobic fitness, it is the ability of the circulatory and respiratory systems to adjust to and recover from the effects of such activities as brisk walking, running, swimming, cycling, and other moderate-to-vigorous activities.
- **Body composition:** the relative amounts of body fat and lean body tissue or fat-free mass (muscle, bone, water, skin, blood, and other nonfat tissues). Body composition is often expressed as percent body fat.
- **Musculoskeletal fitness:**

  **Flexibility:** the ability of the joints to move through a full range of movement (e.g., touching one's toes with legs straight while seated on the floor).

  **Muscular strength:** the maximal one-effort force that can be exerted against a resistance (e.g., lifting the heaviest weight possible in the bench press or leg squat).

  **Muscular endurance:** the ability of the muscles to supply a submaximal force repeatedly (e.g., sit-ups, push-ups, chin-ups, or lifting weights 10 to 15 times in the weight room).

There are many activities that develop components of both skill- and health-related physical fitness. These include basketball, racquetball and handball, ice skating and roller skating, and soccer. Many individuals prefer to play sports while getting fit rather than engaging in "pure" fitness activities like running, cycling, or stair climbing. The competitive and social aspects of sports make them enjoyable for many, and help promote long-lasting compliance (one of the greatest challenges in exercise training).

However, many sports such as baseball, table tennis, golf (with a cart), volleyball, and bowling, while demanding certain athletic skills, do little to promote the components of health-related fitness. This is because they fail to stimulate the heart, lungs, and muscles at a level sufficient to cause positive changes. These sporting activities should be supplemented with fitness routines to ensure long-term health. Athletes who excel in throwing a ball or swinging a golf club should understand that they may not have optimal levels of body fat or cardiorespiratory fitness and as a consequence may be at higher risk for chronic disease. Conversely, though individuals may possess poor coordination and dislike athletic sports, they can still be physically fit and healthy if they engage regularly in aerobic and musculoskeletal exercise.

Each of the components of health-related fitness can be measured separately from the others, and specific exercises have been fashioned to develop each of the areas. These will be reviewed later in this chapter. The important point here is that "total fitness" is equated with the development of each of the major components through a well-rounded exercise program. Some individuals weight train to develop muscular strength and endurance but pay little attention to aerobic exercise for their cardiorespiratory system. Some runners rank high in heart and lung fitness but low in upper-body strength.

There are some modes of exercise that "do it all," such as rowing, cross-country skiing, swimming, and aerobic dance, which train both the upper- and lower-body musculature while giving the heart and lung system a good workout. Table 1.1 rates various activities according to their overall potential for developing "total fitness."

Individuals who engage in regular physical activity to develop cardiorespiratory endurance, musculoskeletal fitness, and optimal body fat levels improve their basic energy levels and place themselves at lower risk for heart disease, cancer, diabetes, osteoporosis, and other chronic diseases. Scientific evidence supporting this perspective will be reviewed throughout the rest of this book. In accordance with this viewpoint, the American College of Sports Medicine (ACSM) has de- fined health-related physical fitness as "a state characterized by an ability to perform daily activities with vigor and a demonstration of traits and capacities that are associated with low risk of premature development of the hypokinetic diseases (i.e., those associated with physical inactivity)."

Physically fit individuals can accomplish the ordinary tasks of life (e.g., carrying groceries, climbing stairs, gardening) with less fatigue, storing up an energy reserve for leisure-time exercise or unforeseen emergencies. As summarized by Dr. Harrison Clarke, one of America's most noted fitness leaders during the 1960s, "Physical fitness is the ability to last, to bear up, to withstand stress, and to persevere under difficult circumstances where an unfit person would give up. Physical fitness is the opposite to being fatigued from ordinary efforts, to lacking the energy to enter zestfully into life's activities, and to becoming exhausted from unexpected, demanding physical exertion."

## Cardiorespiratory Fitness

Cardiorespiratory endurance or aerobic fitness is enhanced when large muscle masses of the body are involved in continuous and rhythmic

## TABLE 1.1
## Fitness Benefits of Selected Physical Activities

Activities are rated on a 5-point scale in terms of their capacity to develop aerobic fitness/body composition (these are grouped together because they both deal with energy expenditure) or muscular strength/endurance. 1 = not at all; 2 = somewhat or just a little; 3 = moderately; 4 = strongly; 5 = very strongly. For muscular strength and endurance, the activity is rated high if both upper- and lower-body musculature are improved. In general, activities that rank high in aerobic fitness/body composition would also rank high in chronic disease prevention. *Author's choice for best overall modes of physical activity for total fitness.

| Physical activity | Aerobic fitness and body composition | Muscular strength and endurance |
|---|---|---|
| *Aerobic dance, moderate to hard | 4 | 4 |
| Basketball, game play | 4 | 2 |
| Bicycling, fast pace | 5 | 3 |
| *Canoeing, rowing, hard pace | 5 | 4 |
| Circuit weight training | 3 | 5 |
| Handball, game play | 4 | 3 |
| Golf, walking, carrying bag | 3 | 2 |
| Lawn mowing, power push | 3 | 3 |
| Racquetball, squash, game play | 4 | 3 |
| Rope jumping, moderate to hard | 4 | 3 |
| Running, brisk pace | 5 | 2 |
| Rollerblading/skating | 4 | 3 |
| *Shoveling dirt, digging | 4 | 4 |
| Skiing, downhill | 2 | 3 |
| *Skiing, cross-country | 5 | 4 |
| Soccer | 4 | 3 |
| *Splitting wood | 4 | 4 |
| Stair climbing | 5 | 3 |
| *Swimming | 5 | 4 |
| Tennis, game play | 3 | 3 |
| Volleyball, game play | 3 | 3 |
| Walking, briskly | 3 | 2 |
| Weight training | 2 | 5 |

activity for at least three to five exercise sessions a week, 20-60 minutes a session, at an intensity of 50-85 percent $\dot{V}O_2$max. Typical aerobic activities include running, swimming, cycling, brisk walking, and various vigorous sports. Cardiorespiratory endurance is considered health related because low levels have been consistently linked with a markedly increased risk of premature death from most of the major causes of death.

In 1968, Dr. Kenneth H. Cooper published his book *Aerobics,* which ignited a worldwide interest in cardiorespiratory or aerobic fitness. In this book, Cooper challenged Americans to take personal charge of their lifestyles by engaging in regular aerobic exercise to counter the epidemics of heart disease, obesity, and rising health care costs.

Cooper emphasized that the best form of exercise is "aerobic," a word he coined to represent activities that train the heart, lungs, and blood vessels. Stated Cooper, "The best exercises are running, swimming, cycling, walking, stationary running, handball, basketball, and squash, and in just about that order. . . . Isometrics, weight lifting, and calisthenics, though good as far as they go, don't even make the list, despite the fact that most exercise books are based on one of these three, especially calisthenics."

Millions took up the "aerobic challenge" and began jogging, cycling, walking, and swimming their way to better health. The running boom, the aerobic dance movement, and a surge in the health and fitness club industry followed in quick order. Before the release of Cooper's book, most fitness leaders had emphasized the development of muscular strength and size because little was known about the importance of aerobic fitness to health and longevity.

According to the ACSM, cardiorespiratory endurance is considered health related because people who avoid aerobic exercise have been consistently linked with a markedly increased risk of premature death from all causes, especially heart disease. Chapters to follow in this book will review scientific evidence supporting the idea that aerobically fit individuals have a lower risk for coronary heart disease, stroke, various types of cancer, diabetes, high blood pressure, obesity, osteoporosis, depression, and anxiety.

Having good cardiorespiratory endurance is exemplified by such characteristics as the ability to run, cycle, or swim for prolonged periods of time. When the large muscle masses of the body are involved in continuous and rhythmic activity, the circulatory and respiratory systems increase their activity to provide sufficient oxygen to burn fuel to provide energy for the working muscles.

In the laboratory, the ability of the body to take in oxygen, transport it, and use it to burn fuel can be measured with cycle ergometers or treadmills and a metabolic cart. The person being tested exercises to an ever increasing workload while the metabolic cart uses oxygen and carbon dioxide analyzers combined with measurement of ventilation to calculate $\dot{V}O_2$max.

$\dot{V}O_2$max, or maximal aerobic power, is defined as the greatest rate at which oxygen can be consumed during maximal exercise; it is typically expressed in terms of milliliters of oxygen consumed per kilogram of body weight per minute ($ml \cdot kg^{-1} \cdot min^{-1}$). When body weight is factored in, it becomes possible to compare the $\dot{V}O_2max$ of people of varying size in different environments.

Laboratory measurement of $\dot{V}O_2max$ is expensive and requires highly trained personnel. Various tests (such as the 1.5-mile run or 1-mile walk test) have been developed as substitutes that allow people to estimate their $\dot{V}O_2max$ with some degree of accuracy.

The fittest athletes in the world range in $\dot{V}O_2max$ from 65 to 94 $ml \cdot kg^{-1} \cdot min^{-1}$ and include cross-country skiers, long-distance runners, and cyclists. "Good" levels for adult men are above 45 $ml \cdot kg^{-1} \cdot min^{-1}$ (equivalent to running a mile in under eight minutes), and for adult women, 40 $ml \cdot kg^{-1} \cdot min^{-1}$ (a mile in under nine minutes).

To improve cardiorespiratory endurance or $\dot{V}O_2max$, ACSM recommends that the basic aerobic program be conducted three to five times a week, 20-60 minutes per session, at an intensity of 50-85 percent $\dot{V}O_2max$ (or 60-90 percent of the maximal heart rate). As the frequency, duration, and intensity are increased, greater gains in $\dot{V}O_2max$ will be experienced. When improvement of health alone is the goal, lower-intensity physical activity spread throughout the day appears sufficient. This will be discussed in greater detail later in this chapter.

## Body Composition

Body composition is the ratio of fat to fat-free weight and is often expressed as percent body fat. Healthy body fat percentages fall under 15 percent for men and 23 percent for women. Obesity, defined as the excessive accumulation of body fat, has been linked to most of the major diseases that afflict modern men and women. The obese people most vulnerable to disease have android or apple-shaped obesity as compared to the safer gynoid or pear-shaped obesity. Many methods such as skinfold testing and underwater weighing have been developed to measure body fat; these provide a much better estimate of ideal body weight than do height-weight tables.

Body weight can be divided into fat and fat-free weight. The fat-free weight is primarily muscle, bone, and water. Percent body fat, which is the percentage of total weight represented by fat weight, is the preferred index used to evaluate a person's body composition. Figure 1.3 shows healthy and unhealthy levels of percent body fat.

Research to establish ways of determining body fat percentage began during the 1940s. Since then, a wide variety of methods have been used, including underwater weighing, skinfold testing, bioelectrical

**Men**

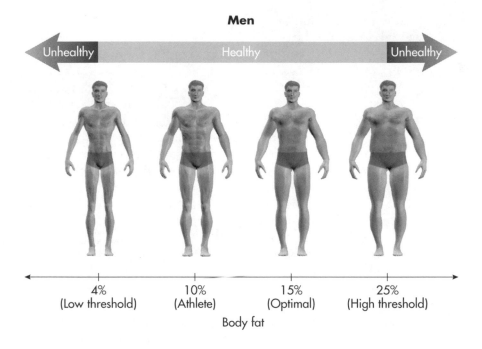

| 4% | 10% | 15% | 25% |
| (Low threshold) | (Athlete) | (Optimal) | (High threshold) |

Body fat

**Women**

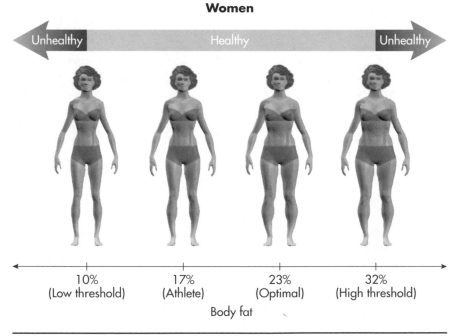

| 10% | 17% | 23% | 32% |
| (Low threshold) | (Athlete) | (Optimal) | (High threshold) |

Body fat

FIGURE 1.3    Ideal body fat percentages fall under 15 percent for men and 23 percent for women.

impedance, infrared interactance, dual-energy x-ray absorptiometry, and computed tomography.

Height-weight tables present weight ranges that are recommended for a given height, but they provide only a rough estimate of one's ideal or healthy body weight. People vary widely in their fat-free weight, such that muscular and athletic individuals are usually defined as "overweight" according to the height-weight tables despite having low amounts of body fat. At the same time, those with small amounts of muscle and bone can often be designated as "underweight" when in actuality they may be carrying too much body fat. For these reasons, it is recommended that concerned individuals have their body fat measured at a reputable health and fitness facility to gain a true picture of their body fat percentage and ideal body weight.

Interest in measurement of body composition has grown tremendously during the last 20 years, largely because of the relationship of body composition to both health and athletic performance. Later in this book (part II), recent scientific data linking obesity with coronary heart disease, several types of cancer, stroke, diabetes, osteoarthritis, high blood cholesterol, and high blood pressure will be reviewed. Many health experts believe that next to avoidance of smoking, keeping the body fat at an optimal level is one of the most important goals in staying healthy and avoiding disease.

Recent information is showing that with respect to medical complications, it makes a difference where the excess fat is deposited. The obese people most vulnerable to disease tend to have more of their fat deposited in abdominal areas rather than in the hip and thigh areas. In other words, health risks are greater for those who have much of their body fat in the upper body, especially the trunk and abdominal areas. This is called android obesity (or apple shaped) in comparison to gynoid obesity (or pear shaped, characterized by deposition of fat in the hips and thighs).

The ratio of waist and hip circumferences (WHR) is a simple and convenient method of determining the type of obesity present. The risk of disease increases strongly when the WHR of men rises above 0.9, and that of women, above 0.8. In other words, when the waist circumference is nearly the same size as or greater than the hip circumference, android obesity is diagnosed, which predicts greater-than-normal disease complications from obesity.

## Muscular Strength and Endurance

To develop muscular size, strength, and endurance, a minimum resistance training program is two sessions per week in which the weight trainer lifts one set, 8 to 12 repetitions of 8 to 10 different exercises that train all of the major muscle groups. Health benefits associated with resistance training include improved bone density, muscular size and strength, and connective tissue strength as well as a lowering of the risk for low back pain, osteoporosis, and frailty in old age. Development of muscular strength and endurance has not been consistently linked with lowered risk of heart disease, cancer, diabetes, or other chronic diseases and does not appreciably improve aerobic fitness.

As stated earlier, muscular strength is the maximum one-effort force that a person can generate against a resistance, while muscular endurance is the ability of the muscles to repeat a submaximal effort over and over.

The ACSM recommends that individuals who desire basic muscular strength and endurance lift weights at least twice a week, engaging in a minimum of one set, 8 to 12 repetitions of 8 to 10 different exercises that involve all of the major muscle groups. Although this "beginner" program may help to develop and maintain muscular strength, endurance, and size, three or five sessions per week using three or more sets of a wide variety of weight-lifting exercises are recommended for optimal gains.

Development of muscular strength and endurance has several important health-related benefits, including increased bone density (lowering risk of osteoporosis), muscle size, and connective tissue strength and improved self-esteem. Between the ages of 30 and 70, muscle size and strength decrease by an average of 30 percent, much of this due to inactivity. This contributes to the weakness and frailty common in old age. According to recent studies, elderly people who train with weights can recapture a good portion of their lost strength, enabling them to better perform the common daily activities of life.

Low back pain has been related to weak spinal and abdominal muscles. During certain types of lifting or exercise, weak trunk muscles may be unable to support the spine properly, leading to low back pain. Intensive back muscle exercise programs provide excellent therapy for people who have low back pain, helping to reduce their pain and enabling them to return to work earlier than would otherwise be expected.

There is little evidence to suggest that weight lifting reduces the risk for heart disease, cancer, diabetes, hypertension, high blood cholesterol, or other chronic diseases and risk factors. Training with weights does not increase the $\dot{V}O_2max$ appreciably, primarily because oxygen consumption seldom exceeds 60 percent of $\dot{V}O_2max$. Thus weight lifters should supplement their resistance training with aerobic training.

Many tests have been developed to measure muscular strength and endurance. Some of these use very sophisticated equipment, but good results can be obtained with the use of common tests such as push-ups, chin-ups, sit-ups, the hand-grip test, and the one-repetition bench press test. As a point of reference, it is considered "good" for adult men to do 25 or more push-ups and for adult women to do 20 or more push-ups (adapted with the knees on the ground). For bent-knee sit-ups, the "good" standard is 30 or more within one minute for men, and 25 or more for women.

## Flexibility

Flexibility, or joint range of motion, can be developed using static stretching exercises. At a minimum, three sessions a week are recommended with stretched positions held for 10 to 30 seconds, three to five times, for each major joint. Although many health benefits have been claimed for development of flexibility, few have been supported in well-designed studies. Many sports medicine physicians still recommend flexibility exercises because their clinical experience has shown benefits in preventing injury and treating low back pain.

Flexibility or range of joint motion is specific to each joint of the body. Muscles, ligaments, and tendons influence the amount of movement possible at each joint. Some people are more flexible because these tissues are "looser" around the joint, while in others they are tighter, limiting full range of motion.

The ACSM recommends that static stretching exercises (i.e., stretched positions that are held) be sustained for 10 to 30 seconds, and then be repeated three to five times, for each major joint of the body. At a minimum, three sessions per week are recommended for developing flexibility. As a matter of safety and effectiveness, an active aerobic warm-up should precede vigorous stretching sessions. Muscles that are warm from jogging, cycling, or other aerobic exercise can stretch further and more safely.

Many claims have been made for health-related benefits of flexibility. These include good joint mobility, increased resistance to muscle injury and soreness, lowered risk of low back pain and other spinal column aches and pains, improved posture, more graceful body movements, improved personal appearance and self-image, enhanced development of sport skills, and reduced tension and stress. For example, it has long been held that tight lower back and hamstring muscles combined with weak abdominal and trunk muscles allow the pelvis to tilt forward, increasing the risk of lower back pain.

Unfortunately, there are few convincing studies to support these beliefs. For example, in studies with adolescents and adults, good flexibility has not been able to predict decreased risk of low back pain. Nonetheless, flexibility exercises are included in most low back treatment programs because clinical experience has shown that they appear to help.

Regarding injury potential, in one study of soccer players there was found to be no relationship between past injuries and muscle tightness. In another study of gymnasts, those with greater toe-touching ability actually had more back pain than their "tighter" teammates. More research is needed to sort out the true benefits related to flexibility training. Most sports medicine specialists still recommend stretching to prevent injuries because their clinical experience has shown this practice to be beneficial.

Flexibility is related to age and physical activity. As a person ages, flexibility decreases, although this is thought to be due more to inactivity than to the aging process itself.

One of the standard tests for hamstring and lower back flexibility is the sit-and-reach test. To perform this test, the individual holds the legs straight with the feet flat against a box and attempts to reach as far as possible beyond the foot line. It is considered "good" to reach four or more inches beyond the foot line, with seven or more inches rated as "excellent."

# EXERCISE GUIDELINES FOR IMPROVING HEALTH

Two sets of exercise guidelines have been formulated for two different sets of goals. When the development of cardiorespiratory endurance and health are the objectives, the intensity of exercise training should range between 50 and 85 percent of $\dot{V}O_2$max and should be for 20 to 60 minutes, three to five days a week. When improvement in health is the only goal, the intensity can drop below 50 percent $\dot{V}O_2$max, with 30 minutes or more of physical activity accumulated over the course of most days of the week. This less formal approach to exercise should appeal to a greater number of adults.

During this century, many opinions as to the best type of exercise for the American public have gained favor. As noted earlier in this chapter, during the first half of the century, for example, muscular strength was emphasized by many fitness leaders as the primary goal of an exercise program. During the boom years of the aerobic movement in the 1970s and 1980s, development of cardiorespiratory fitness through high-intensity aerobic exercise was emphasized, often to the detriment of musculoskeletal fitness. The focus of the early 1990s has been on a comprehensive approach to physical fitness in which three major components—cardiorespiratory fitness, musculoskeletal fitness, and body composition—are given balanced attention.

In 1993, ACSM released its "exercise lite" recommendations, which caught some off guard with their emphasis on general physical activity and disease prevention (see table 1.2). As emphasized earlier in this chapter, when the development of cardiorespiratory endurance is the objective, the intensity of training should range between 50 and 85 percent of $\dot{V}O_2$max (or 60 to 90 percent of maximum heart rate). (The maximum heart rate is defined as the highest heart rate that one can

## TABLE 1.2
## "Exercise Lite"—Physical Activity and Public Health: A Recommendation From the Centers for Disease Control and Prevention and the American College of Sports Medicine—Key Statements

• The current low participation rate may be due in part to the misperception of many people that to reap health benefits they must engage in vigorous, continuous exercise. The scientific evidence clearly demonstrates that regular, moderate-intensity physical activity provides substantial health benefits.

• Every U.S. adult should accumulate 30 minutes or more of moderate-intensity physical activity on most, preferably all, days of the week. . . . One way to meet this standard is to walk two miles briskly. . . .

• Intermittent activity also confers substantial benefits. Therefore, the recommended 30 minutes of activity can be accumulated in short bouts of activity: walking up the stairs instead of taking the elevator, walking instead of driving short distances, doing calisthenics, or pedaling a stationary cycle while watching television.

• The health benefits gained from increased physical activity depend on the initial physical activity level. Sedentary individuals are expected to benefit most from increasing their activity to the recommended level.

• Two other components of fitness—flexibility and muscular strength—should not be overlooked. Clinical experience and limited studies suggest that people who maintain or improve their strength and flexibility may be better able to perform daily activities, may be less likely to develop back pain, and may be better able to avoid disability, especially as they advance into older age.

• If Americans who lead sedentary lives would adopt a more active lifestyle, there would be enormous benefit to the public's health and to individual well-being. An active lifestyle does not require a regimented, vigorous exercise program. Instead, small changes that increase daily physical activity will enable individuals to reduce their risk of chronic disease and may contribute to enhanced quality of life.

Source: Pate, R.R, Pratt, M., Blair, S.N., et al. (1995). Physical activity and public health. *JAMA* 273:402-407.

achieve during maximal exercise.) When improvement in health is of more concern, the intensity can drop below 50 percent, and people in the general population are simply urged to "accumulate 30 minutes or more of moderate-intensity physical activity over the course of most days of the week." These recommendations from ACSM complement each other, and people should adapt them in accordance with their own personal goals.

The important point, according to ACSM, is that "if Americans who lead sedentary lives would adopt a more active lifestyle, there would be enormous benefit to the public's health and to individual well-being. An active lifestyle does not require a regimented, vigorous exercise program. Instead, small changes that increase daily physical activity will enable individuals to reduce their risk of chronic disease and may contribute to enhanced quality of life."

In summary, a "total fitness" approach ensures that the heart and lungs and all of the major muscle groups are developed while the joints are kept flexible and body fat is maintained at a healthy level. Another goal in keeping the body fit is to enhance overall health and decrease the risk for heart disease, cancer, and other common diseases. While the health goal can be reached through regular moderate physical activity, a program of vigorous exercise is needed to develop physical fitness.

# REFERENCES

American College of Sports Medicine. (1995). *Guidelines for graded exercise testing and prescription.* Philadelphia: Lea & Febiger.

Caspersen, C.J., & Merritt, R.K. (1995). Physical activity trends among 26 states, 1986-1990. *Medicine and Science in Sports and Exercise, 27*, 713-720.

Cooper, K.H. (1968). *Aerobics.* New York: Bantam Books.

King, A.C. (1994). Community and public health approaches to the promotion of physical activity. *Medicine and Science in Sports and Exercise, 26*, 1405-1412.

McGinnis, J.M., & Lee, P.R. (1995). *Healthy People 2000* at mid decade. *Journal of the American Medical Association, 273*, 1123-1129.

Nieman, D.C. (1994). The exercise test as a component of the total fitness evaluation. *Primary Care, 21*, 569-587.

Nieman, D.C. (1995). *Fitness and sports medicine: A health-related approach.* Mountain View, CA: Mayfield.

Pate, R.R., Pratt, M., Blair, S.N., et al. (1995). Physical activity and public health: A recommendation from the Centers for Disease Control and Prevention and the American College of Sports Medicine. *Journal of the American Medical Association, 273*, 402-407.

U.S. Department of Health and Human Services. (1996). *Physical activity and health: A report of the Surgeon General.* Atlanta: U.S. Department of Health and Human Services, Centers for Disease Control and Prevention, National Center for Chronic Disease Prevention and Health Promotion.

# Chapter 2

# HOW THE BODY ADAPTS TO EXERCISE

*Lack of activity destroys the good condition of every human being while movement and methodical physical exercise save and preserve it.*

Plato

The human body is designed for action. The elongated muscle groups, tendons, and ligaments allow the arms and legs to engage in a wide variety of work and sport activities, while the brain coordinates delivery of blood, oxygen, and fuel from the heart and lungs. All of the various systems of the body communicate with one another through chemical and nervous pathways to ensure a precise coordination of activity. The more these systems are used, the easier and more enjoyable exercise becomes. In contrast, lack of movement, as Plato cautioned, leads to feebleness and poor condition. In this chapter, the major benefits of exercise training on the human body will be outlined, with consideration given to the influence of genetics, gender, and age.

## EFFECTS OF EXERCISE ON THE BODY

During one aerobic exercise bout of 30 to 45 minutes, the rate of breathing increases approximately three times above resting levels, while the amount of air entering the lungs is 20 times higher. The heart rate doubles or triples, the volume of blood pumped out of the heart increases four- to sixfold, and the oxygen consumed by the working muscles of the body climbs more than 10 times above resting levels.

These sudden, temporary changes in body function caused by exercise are called acute responses to exercise, and they disappear shortly after the exercise period is finished.

If the aerobic exercise sessions are continued nearly daily for at least several weeks, body function starts to change during both rest and exercise. The resting heart rate slows 10 to 30 beats per minute, and during any given exercise workload, the heart beats more slowly because it is a more efficient pump. The exercising heart can pump out more blood with each beat, and the lungs can ventilate more air when challenged with high-intensity exercise. The net result is that more oxygen is delivered to the muscles, allowing them to burn more fuel and produce more energy for exercise (i.e., enhanced metabolism). $\dot{V}O_2$max, the maximum amount of oxygen that can be consumed by the body at the point of maximal exertion, increases markedly. The muscles themselves become more efficient in storing and burning fats and carbohydrates.

Figure 2.1 summarizes the intimate link between ventilation, circulation, and metabolism. Trained individuals experience enhancement in each area as the lungs, heart and blood vessels, and muscles adapt to improve oxygen delivery and energy production for exercise performance.

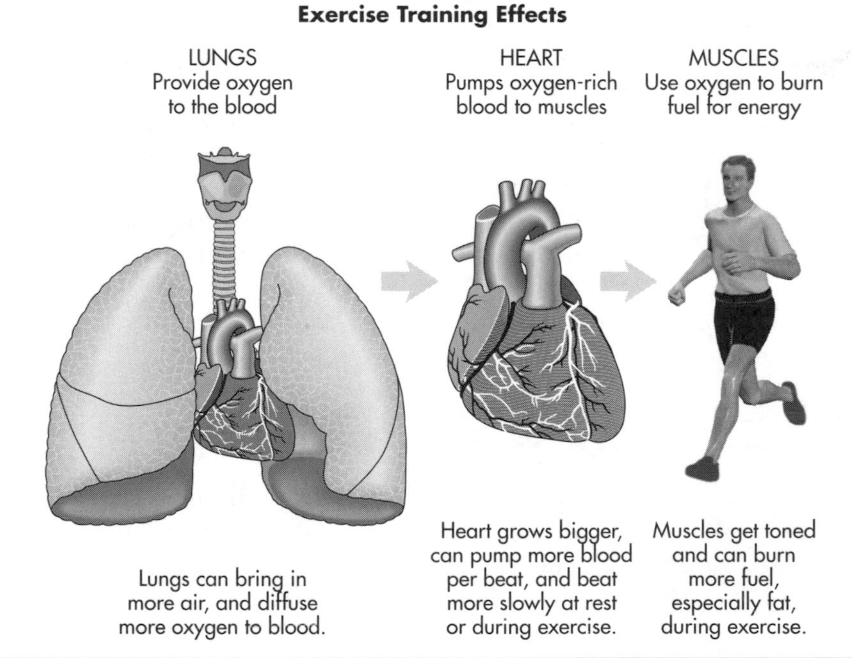

## Exercise Training Effects

| LUNGS | HEART | MUSCLES |
|---|---|---|
| Provide oxygen to the blood | Pumps oxygen-rich blood to muscles | Use oxygen to burn fuel for energy |

| Lungs can bring in more air, and diffuse more oxygen to blood. | Heart grows bigger, can pump more blood per beat, and beat more slowly at rest or during exercise. | Muscles get toned and can burn more fuel, especially fat, during exercise. |
|---|---|---|

FIGURE 2.1   Ventilation, circulation, and metabolism are intimately linked, and each improves with training.

These persistent changes in the structure and function of the body following regular exercise training are called chronic adaptations to exercise—changes that enable to the body to respond more easily to exercise. Many of these changes occur rapidly. For example, within the first one to three weeks of intensive aerobic exercise training, significant improvements in $\dot{V}O_2$max, resting and exercise heart rate, and lung ventilation can be measured. Some adaptations to aerobic exercise take longer. For example, the increase in the number of blood capillaries (the smallest blood vessels) within the muscle may take months and years.

The magnitude of the chronic changes depends on the amount and intensity of exercise, as well as the initial fitness status. For example, overweight and middle-aged people who have been inactive for many years have the potential to improve $\dot{V}O_2$max by nearly 100 percent, while college students can expect smaller gains (about 10 to 20 percent). Those engaging in a moderate walking program will not experience the same gains in heart and lung function that runners will.

Interestingly, exercise-induced changes in body function are lost just as rapidly as they are gained. In this chapter, both the acute and chronic adaptations will be clarified, with an emphasis on regular exercise training to avoid quick reversals in fitness (termed "detraining").

As emphasized in the previous chapter, improvements in health can be expected with *both* moderate and intensive aerobic training programs. Each individual will have to decide what is most important to him or her—health, aerobic fitness, or both. Other than the health benefits, a high aerobic fitness level allows people to engage in vigorous outdoor recreational activities and perform more successfully in most individual, dual, and team sports.

## The Heart

The single biggest difference between endurance-trained and untrained individuals is the size of the stroke volume, or the amount of blood pumped out of the heart each beat. With exercise training, the heart gets bigger and stronger. As a result, the resting heart rate is slower in trained individuals, while during exercise a given amount of blood output can be achieved at a lower heart rate. The net result is that trained people can run, swim, and cycle faster because the heart is capable of a greater blood output, delivering more oxygen to the working muscles.

The heart, about the size of the human fist, pumps about five liters of blood through 60,000 miles of blood vessels each minute at rest. Since the average adult body contains about five liters of blood, nearly all of it passes through the heart each minute. The resting heart rate of most untrained humans is 60 to 80 beats per minute, and 55 to 75 milliliters of blood is pumped out of the heart with each beat (defined as the stroke volume).

The cardiac output (the amount of blood pumped out of the heart each minute) is simply the number of heart beats times the amount of blood pumped out with each beat. So in an individual with a resting heart rate of 70 beats per minute and a stroke volume of 70 milliliters per minute, the total cardiac output is 70 bpm × 70 ml/min or 4,900 milliliters of blood per minute.

With regular aerobic exercise training, the heart gets bigger and stronger. In fact, one of the most important differences between un-trained and trained individuals is the size of the heart and its ability to pump out more blood during exercise. At one time, the increase in heart size was thought to be harmful to one's health (i.e., the so-called athlete's heart). This is now recognized as a normal and beneficial change that occurs with regular aerobic exercise.

The left ventricle, which pumps out blood from the heart to the body, undergoes the greatest increase in size. What this means is that at rest, the trained and larger heart pumps out more blood per beat (i.e., has a larger stroke volume). For example, while sedentary people have stroke volumes at rest of about 60 milliliters, those of athletes often measure greater than 100 milliliters.

The larger stroke volume allows the heart to pump more slowly. The resting heart rate decreases approximately one beat per minute for 1 to 2 weeks of aerobic training, for about 10 to 20 weeks. Further decreases are possible if training duration and intensity are increased. Many of the world's best endurance athletes have resting heart rates below 40 beats per minute. For example, Miguel Indurain, one of the best cyclists in history, had a resting heart rate of 28 beats per minute.

The heart rate during exercise increases in direct proportion to the level of exercise intensity. The maximum heart rate is the highest heart rate that can be measured at the point of exhaustion during an all-out effort. Subtracting age from 220 gives a rough estimation of an indivi-dual's maximum heart rate. For example, a 40-year-old is estimated to have a maximum heart rate of 180 beats per minute (220 – 40 = 180).

The American College of Sports Medicine recommends that people exercise at 60 to 90 percent of their maximum heart rate to achieve a beneficial effect on their cardiorespiratory system. For a 40-year-old individual, this would be 108 to 162 beats per minute, with the higher end of the range producing greater training benefits. Of interest to people who measure their heart rates during exercise is that as the weeks of training pass by, a faster speed is necessary to achieve the same heart rate. In other words, because the heart gets larger and stronger, it can pump more blood and oxygen, meaning that it can accomplish the same work at a lower heart rate. To keep the heart rate at the proper intensity, the trained exerciser will have to run, cycle, or swim faster to achieve a continued training effect.

The trained individual also experiences an increase in the total amount of blood in the body. Sedentary people have about five liters of blood and elite athletes close to six liters, while trained individuals fall somewhere in between.

During exercise, blood is diverted away from areas where it is not needed (i.e., intestinal organs) to the muscles. At rest, only one-fifth of the blood output from the heart goes to the muscles, as compared to three-fourths during heavy aerobic exercise. With regular exercise, the body does a better job at shutting down blood vessels in inactive areas and opening up those in active muscle areas. To look at this another way, the blood vessels, which are made up primarily of muscle, also become fit with exercise, and can constrict and dilate better to channel the blood to where it is most needed.

As the body heats up during exercise, an increasing amount of blood is directed to the skin where fluid is given up to produce sweat. At the same time, the blood gives up fluid to the muscles to help them contract and work better. The net result is that the blood gets thicker. Obviously, having more blood means that the athlete is better equipped to share blood fluid with both the muscles and skin, enhancing performance.

The blood carries oxygen to the working muscles where it is used to burn carbohydrates and fats, providing energy for exercise. As the heart gets bigger and stronger with regular exercise training, more blood can be pumped out during heavy or maximal exercise, increasing the oxygen delivery to the muscle (i.e., $\dot{V}O_2$max is enhanced). As will be discussed later in this chapter, aerobically trained muscles can extract and use oxygen at a higher rate than can untrained muscles. So the higher $\dot{V}O_2$max found among the trained is due primarily to two factors: a greater heart blood output and a greater oxygen extraction by the muscle cells.

As described previously, $\dot{V}O_2$max typically increases 10 to 20 percent with training; higher gains are experienced by overweight and unfit people who lose weight and train long and hard. The highest $\dot{V}O_2$max values have been measured in elite endurance athletes such as cross-country skiers and long-distance runners. These individuals often have $\dot{V}O_2$max values above 80 ml $\cdot$ kg$^{-1}$ $\cdot$ min$^{-1}$ (two times greater than sedentary people), with maximal cardiac outputs greater than 35 liters of blood per minute (compared to less than 20 liters per minute in the sedentary). As will be discussed later, some of these differences between elite athletes and the sedentary have a genetic basis.

# The Lungs

As exercise intensity increases, more and more air must be taken into the lungs to provide oxygen for the working muscles. Although lung size changes little with aerobic exercise training, fit people are capable of ventilating much larger volumes of air during heavy exertion. The lungs, however, are seldom a limiting factor in ability to perform hard aerobic exercise. During moderate-to-hard exercise bouts, aerobically fit individuals are more efficient in transporting and utilizing oxygen, so less air needs to be ventilated by the lungs at a certain exercise workload than for the untrained.

The lungs take in air and pass oxygen to the blood through 300 million tiny "air sacs" known as alveoli. The enormous number of these alveoli provides a surface area equal to that of a tennis court, allowing oxygen to diffuse rapidly into the blood. Also exchanged is carbon dioxide that is produced by the body and then passed to the outside air.

Since ordinary air is only about 21 percent oxygen, the lungs must take in large amounts of air during exercise to supply enough oxygen for the working muscles. Most humans at rest need 250 milliliters of oxygen each minute for life to continue. This oxygen can be supplied by breathing in about six liters of air per minute.

During heavy exercise, oxygen consumption by the body increases 10- to 20-fold or higher, depending on the person's fitness level. This requires 100 to 200 liters of air per minute. Tall and highly trained endurance athletes can have maximal lung ventilation rates in excess of 240 liters per minute, twice the rate found in untrained people. The fitter a person is, the more air the individual can bring into the lungs at maximal exercise—a huge advantage when high-end performance is the goal.

At rest, the normal person breathes 12 times a minute, bringing in one-half liter of air per breath, or six liters per minute. During maximal exercise, the frequency of breathing in athletes is about 55 to 60 breaths a minute, with more than three liters of air taken in each breath. Untrained people cannot breathe this fast or bring in as much air per breath.

Interestingly, with exercise training, lung size changes little. The amount of air breathed in during rest also changes little with training. But during a submaximal exercise bout (i.e., a normal training session at a certain speed), the amount of air ventilated is lower in trained people. In other words, trained people can ventilate less air while achieving the same oxygen intake and exercise workload. The trained body is more efficient in transporting and utilizing oxygen, so less air is required per unit of oxygen consumed. This provides a ventilation reserve that can be used for heavy aerobic exertion.

The oxygen content per unit of blood actually changes very little with aerobic exercise training. The increase in blood volume that comes with training is primarily due to an increase in the fluid portion (i.e., the plasma volume). Red blood cells, which actually transport the oxygen from the lungs to the working muscles, do increase in number; but the gain in plasma volume is typically much higher, resulting in a more fluid blood. The trained person does have more blood, however, which means that the total amount of oxygen actually in the blood increases somewhat.

Overall, the lungs are quite proficient in bringing adequate amounts of oxygen into the body. For this reason, the lungs are seldom a limiting factor in ability to perform intense aerobic exercise. The heart is more of a "weak link," because the job of pumping enough blood to the working muscles is a difficult one. Studies have shown that the lungs and muscles can both handle more blood and oxygen than the heart is capable of pumping.

## The Skeletal Muscles

Although the heart appears to be the limiting factor during acute intense aerobic exercise, as the weeks go by and changes take place in the cardiorespiratory system, further improvement in $\dot{V}O_2$max becomes more and more dependent on changes taking place in the muscles themselves. The aerobically trained muscle has more capillaries, fuel (both carbohydrate, or glycogen, and fat), mitochondria (power components in the cells) and energy-producing enzymes, and myoglobin (which stores and shuttles oxygen from the blood to the mitochondria). Aerobic exercise training primarily increases the size of slow-twitch muscle fibers, while strength training increases the size of fast-twitch fibers. People are born with a certain ratio of slow-twitch to fast-twitch muscle fibers, and exercise training does little to alter it.

Experts have debated for decades whether aerobic exercise-induced changes in the heart and lungs are more important to improvement in fitness than changes that take place within the muscles. There is a growing consensus that the heart appears to be the limiting factor during acute intense aerobic exercise. However, as the weeks go by and changes take place in the cardiorespiratory system, further improvement in $\dot{V}O_2$max becomes more and more dependent on changes taking place within the muscles themselves.

In response to regular aerobic training, many significant adaptations take place within the muscle cells. The muscle stores more fuel, both carbohydrates and fats, and develops more enzymes and mitochondria (i.e., energy and power cell components) to burn the fuel more efficiently.

The muscles especially become adept at burning fat for fuel. This is important because fat is more plentiful than carbohydrate (i.e., glycogen). Although it takes more oxygen to burn fat for energy during aerobic exercise, the fit person can supply the extra oxygen, conserving the muscle glycogen that is in shorter supply and is useful during the later stages of long-endurance exercise.

Forms of aerobic exercise such as running, cycling, swimming, and cross-country skiing each rely on the type of muscle cell called slow-twitch fibers. Muscles with a high percentage of slow-twitch fibers are darker than those filled with fast-twitch fibers (which are important for jumping, sprinting, and weight lifting).

With regular aerobic exercise, the slow-twitch fibers increase in size. However, most studies have shown that endurance training does not appreciably change the percentages of slow-twitch and fast-twitch muscle fibers. Each person is born with a certain ratio of slow-twitch and fast-twitch fibers, and little can be done to alter this. Elite endurance athletes usually have a high proportion of slow-twitch fibers, while elite sprinters have a high proportion of fast-twitch fibers. They are born with these high proportions, and then train intensely for years to build up the size of these muscle fibers.

When oxygen enters the muscle cell, it attaches to myoglobin, a pigment that gives slow-twitch fibers their dark appearance. Myoglobin turns red when attached to oxygen and shuttles the oxygen to the mitochondria, which use it to burn fuel and produce energy. Aerobic exercise training can increase muscle myoglobin content by 75 to 80 percent.

One of the most important changes that occur within the muscles with aerobic exercise training is an increase in the number of capillaries surrounding each muscle cell. The presence of more capillaries means that oxygen and fuel delivery, as well as carbon dioxide and heat removal, are easier, improving exercise ability. Capillaries begin to build within the first few months of exercise training, but the network may continue to grow for years in athletes who train intensively.

The changes that occur within the muscle in response to strength training are very different from those just described for aerobic training. Weight lifting leads to an increase in the size of fast-twitch fibers. People who are born with a high percentage of fast-twitch fibers can "bulk up" more easily than those who have mainly slow-twitch fibers. The total protein within the muscle cells increases, and the supporting ligaments, tendons, and other connective tissues all increase in size and strength. Overall, the body's lean body mass (fat-free tissue) increases.

It should be understood that $\dot{V}O_2$max is not significantly improved with weight training. Most experts feel that the majority of weight-lifting exercises involve a relatively small muscle mass exercised intensely for a short period of time. This is called "anaerobic exercise" (i.e., without oxygen) and is valuable for increasing muscle bulk, but not $\dot{V}O_2$max.

Weight lifters often note that their heart rates seems to be elevated during weight-training sessions, but this is due to the stimulation of the nervous system and is not accompanied by a significant and continuous increase in oxygen consumption. Blood pressures can rise to unusually high levels during heavy weight lifting. The heart adapts to this by increasing the thickness of the left ventricle wall without an increase in volume.

# INFLUENCE OF GENETICS ON AEROBIC FITNESS

It is estimated that heredity accounts for between 25 and 50 percent of the variance one finds in $\dot{V}O_2$max among people. Even the ability to improve aerobic fitness through long-term training has a genetic component. Both genetic factors and exercise habits are important in determining $\dot{V}O_2$max, but genetic factors do appear to set boundary limits for what is possible through exercise training.

Aerobic fitness, or $\dot{V}O_2$max, varies widely between people, and genetic factors explain why some people go to the Olympics and some who train just as hard don't. World-class endurance athletes can increase their $\dot{V}O_2$max to over 80 ml $\cdot$ kg$^{-1}$ $\cdot$ min$^{-1}$, and then stop training and still have values higher than well-conditioned but non-elite individuals (e.g., over 65 ml $\cdot$ kg$^{-1}$ $\cdot$ min$^{-1}$).

Dr. Claude Bouchard from Laval University, Quebec, Canada, has compared aerobic fitness in brothers, fraternal twins, and identical twins. He found that the aerobic fitness levels were much closer in identical twins than in fraternal twins or siblings. Dr. Bouchard has concluded that heredity accounts for between 25 and 50 percent of the variance one finds in $\dot{V}O_2$max between people.

Even the ability to improve $\dot{V}O_2$max has been found to have some dependence on heredity. In other words, some people can improve their aerobic fitness more than others because they have genetic factors that favor this.

Both genetic factors and exercise habits influence aerobic fitness. Genetic factors appear to set the upper bounds of what is possible, while hard training pushes fitness up to this upper boundary. Dr. Per-Olaf Åstrand, one of the world's top exercise experts, has emphasized that the best way to become an Olympic champion is to be selective when choosing parents!

# INFLUENCE OF GENDER ON AEROBIC FITNESS

When one compares the best male and female athletes in running and swimming, for example, world record times for women are about 6 to 13 percent slower. Although social and cultural constraints still operate, most experts feel that several biological factors are more important when considering gender differences in performance. Even at the elite athletic level, women, compared with men, have a smaller fat-free mass, greater body fat percentage, lower body strength, smaller heart stroke volume and higher heart rate, lower blood volume and blood hemoglobin content, and lower $\dot{V}O_2$max.

During the last three decades there has been a dramatic increase in the number of women participating in both recreational and competitive sports. With this increase has come a much better understanding of how men and women differ and how they compare in their ability to exercise and compete.

Why are elite female endurance athletes slower than their male counterparts? Is this because of actual biological differences or do the numbers reflect social and cultural constraints? For example, the world marathon record for men is just under 2:07 and for women, just over 2:21—an 11 percent difference. Women, however, have been running the marathon for only about 25 years, whereas men have had the opportunity for nearly four times as long.

Women were prohibited from running any race longer than 800 meters until the 1960s and were barred from official participation in the marathon until 1970. These restrictions were based on the misconception that women were physiologically unqualified for long-endurance activity. Interestingly, in the 1984 Los Angeles Olympics, Joan Benoit ran the first-ever Olympic marathon for women in 2:24:52, a time that would have won 11 of the previous 20 men's Olympic marathons.

Comparison of male and female world records in various running events from the 1970s to the present shows that there were dramatic improvements for women until the mid-1980s, when improvements in women's records leveled off. For distances of 400 meters through the marathon, women's present world records are about 10 to 13 percent slower than men's. Some experts feel that this gender difference will remain because of several biological factors.

Around the time of puberty, major differences in body size, composition, and fitness between males and females begin to emerge. Some of these differences are the following:

- Under the influence of various hormones, especially testosterone, the fat-free mass (i.e., muscle, bone, and other fat-free tissues) increases more in men than in women. By adulthood, the average female has only three-fourths the fat-free mass of men. Women have been found to be 40 to 60 percent weaker than men in upper-body strength and 25 to 30 percent weaker in lower-body strength. Interestingly, for the same amount of muscle, however, there are no differences in strength between men and women. When women lift weights, major increases in strength (20 to 40 percent) can be measured. The gains in strength, however, are related more to neural factors than to increases in muscle size, which tend to be minimal in most women.

- Estrogen in women broadens the pelvis area, stimulates breast development, and increases fat deposition in the thighs and hips. The average adult woman has body fat that is 6 to 10 percentage points above that found in men (e.g., 20 to 25 percent for young adult women compared to 13 to 16 percent for men).

- At a certain relative exercise workload (e.g., 60 percent $\dot{V}O_2max$), the average adult woman has a smaller stroke volume and a higher heart rate than the average man. The lower stroke volume in women appears to be due to their smaller heart size and lower blood volume, both of which are related to the woman's smaller body size. Women also have a lower blood hemoglobin content than men, which means that per unit of blood, less oxygen is available for the working muscles.

- $\dot{V}O_2max$ in the average adult woman is only 70 to 75 percent that of the average man. Some of this difference is attributable to women's relatively lower activity levels. Women do respond to aerobic exercise training similarly to men. But even in elite female endurance athletes, $\dot{V}O_2max$ values are 15 to 30 percent lower than in elite male athletes. A major explanation for this is that even very fit women still carry more body fat than male athletes. If this is adjusted for, the difference between genders falls to about 5 percent.

# INFLUENCE OF AGE ON AEROBIC FITNESS

Increasing evidence supports the contention that a significant proportion of the deterioration attributed to aging can be explained by the tendency of people to exercise less as they age. Although $\dot{V}O_2$max normally declines 8-10 percent per decade after 25 years of age, much of this can be "recaptured" when older people begin regular exercise programs. At any given age, individuals who exercise vigorously can be fitter than their sedentary counterparts, but, because of the aging process, less fit than younger people who exercise. Muscular strength is well preserved to about 45 years of age, but thereafter deteriorates by about 5 to 10 percent per decade. Elderly people respond well to weight training, improving their ability to engage in common daily activities of living.

A key ingredient to healthy aging, according to many gerontologists, is regular physical activity. Of all age groups, elderly people have the most to gain by being active. Yet national surveys indicate that only about one-third of elderly people exercise regularly—less than for any other age group. And recent survey data from the Centers for Disease Control and Prevention indicate that the proportion of elderly people exercising has decreased during the last decade.

Aerobic fitness or $\dot{V}O_2$max normally declines 8 to 10 percent per decade for both males and females after 25 years of age. Nonetheless, at any given age, active people can have a much higher $\dot{V}O_2$max if they exercise vigorously. It has been shown that athletic males and females who are from 65 to 75 years of age can have the $\dot{V}O_2$max of young sedentary adults and that they are capable of performing at levels once thought unattainable.

However, even among athletes who exercise vigorously throughout their lifetimes, $\dot{V}O_2$max still declines at a rate similar to that of sedentary individuals (albeit at a much higher absolute level). Some studies have demonstrated that the rate of decline may be attenuated for several years because of regular, vigorous endurance exercise (with no change in exercise frequency, intensity, or duration), but if subjects are followed long enough, $\dot{V}O_2$max will start falling at normal or accelerated rates.

In other words, the aging process is real, and the ability to exercise intensively is one that diminishes with age. There are no convincing data at this time to show that the age-related decrease in aerobic fitness can be prevented for extended time periods through regular endurance exercise training. A lower heart rate and stroke volume, and lower ability of the muscles to extract oxygen, all appear to contribute to the age-related decline in $\dot{V}O_2$max, even when the individual tries to keep physically active.

The bottom line is that at any given age, athletes who exercise vigorously can be fitter than their sedentary counterparts, but because of the aging process, less fit than younger athletes. Studies have confirmed that peak performance for men is achieved in their 20s for all running and swim events (e.g., 23 years for sprinting and 28 for marathon running).

It should be emphasized, however, that most studies support the concept that untrained people even in their eighth decade of life have not lost the ability to adapt to endurance exercise training. In other words, it is never too late to improve from an untrained to a trained state.

Although earlier studies suggested that older individuals were not as responsive to aerobic training as their younger counterparts, there is now a growing consensus that the relative (but not absolute) increase in $\dot{V}O_2$max over an 8- to 26-week period is similar between young and old adults. In general, the same basic exercise prescription principles used for young adults can be applied to elderly people, but with an emphasis on greater caution and slower progression.

As emphasized earlier, muscular strength in most individuals is well preserved to about 45 years of age, but then deteriorates by about 5 to 10 percent per decade. The average individual will lose about 30 percent of his or her muscle strength and 40 percent of his or her muscle size between the second and seventh decades of life, a process called sarcopenia. This loss in muscle mass appears to be the major reason that strength is decreased among people who are elderly.

In older individuals, muscle weakness may compromise common activities of daily living, leading to dependency on others. Also, reduced leg strength may increase the risk of injury through falling. A growing number of studies have now clearly shown that elderly people are capable of increasing their muscle size and strength in response to weight training. Overall, studies suggest that the rate of decline in strength and muscle mass with increase in age can be curtailed by appropriate resistance training.

# DETRAINING

Detraining, the termination of regular exercise training, causes quick and dramatic changes in cardiovascular fitness, and to a lesser extent, muscular strength and size. After just a few weeks of detraining, aerobic fitness drops significantly as blood volume and stroke volume become smaller. Most of these losses can be avoided by exercising at least three times a week at an intensity of at least 70 percent $\dot{V}O_2$max. After 4 to 12 weeks of no weight training, muscular strength returns to pre-exercise training levels. However, one to two weight-training sessions per week have been shown to be sufficient in maintaining muscular strength.

Physical activity must be continued on a regular basis if one is to retain the benefits to heart, lungs, and muscles. "Use it or lose it" is a proven axiom.

This is especially apparent when subjects undergo long periods of bed rest. In one study conducted by Dr. Bengt Saltin of Sweden, subjects were confined to their beds for 20 days. $VO_2$max dropped 27 percent on average, and the decrease was more pronounced in the fittest subjects. Stroke volume and cardiac blood output each fell 25 percent, due to a decrease in heart and blood volume and the ability of the heart to contract forcibly. It took 10 to 40 days for all subjects to regain their fitness upon retraining.

Most people do not confine themselves to bed when stopping their regular exercise program. Instead, most "detrain," meaning that they cease regular formal exercise training while still going about normal daily work activities.

Dr. Edward Coyle from the University of Texas at Austin has been a leading researcher in the area of detraining. In one study, Dr. Coyle studied the effects of 84 days of no formal exercise on the bodies of athletes who had been training hard for 10 years. Within the first several weeks, runners quickly lost most of their cardiovascular conditioning, highlighted by significant decreases in blood volume, stroke volume, $VO_2$max, muscle glycogen stores, muscle enzymes needed for aerobic exercise, and ability to compete successfully and perform intense aerobic exercise. The number of capillaries in the muscles, however, changed little, even after 84 days of no formal exercise.

In other words, after a person quits regular training, the body loses many of the benefits quickly. Interestingly, most of these losses can be avoided if a person exercises at least three times a week at an intensity of at least 70 percent $VO_2$max. The most important variable here is intensity. In one study of distance runners, when training volume was decreased by more than half during a three-week period while intensity was maintained, no decrement in 5K race performance was experienced.

When a broken limb is immobilized in a rigid cast, muscles quickly lose their size and strength. Within only a few days, the loss in muscle size can be noticed as the cast becomes loose. After several weeks, a large space between the cast and limb indicates that significant muscle wasting or atrophy has occurred.

Detraining also has a strong effect in reducing muscle strength and size. After 4 to 12 weeks of no weight training, muscular strength returns to pre-exercise training levels. However, one to two weight-training sessions per week has been shown to be sufficient in maintaining muscular strength. In other words, once a desired level of muscular strength has been achieved, less effort is needed to maintain it.

In summary, the heart, lungs, and muscles respond readily to a regular regimen of vigorous exercise. Although aerobic fitness is influenced by genetics, gender, and age, each individual can attain a fitness level that meets personal performance goals while making the tasks of daily life easier and more enjoyable.

# REFERENCES

American College of Sports Medicine. (1993). *Resource manual for guidelines for exercise testing and prescription* (2nd ed.). Philadelphia: Lea & Febiger.

Baechle, T.R. (1994). *Essentials of strength training and conditioning.* Champaign, IL: Human Kinetics.

Bouchard, C., Shephard, R.J., & Stephens, T. (1994). *Physical activity, fitness, and health: International proceedings and consensus statement.* Champaign, IL: Human Kinetics.

Houmard, J.A. (1991). Impact of reduced training on performance in endurance athletes. *Sports Medicine, 12,* 380-393.

Nieman, D.C. (1995). *Fitness and sports medicine: A health-related approach.* Palo Alto, CA: Bull.

Rogers, M.A., & Evans, W.J. (1993). Changes in skeletal muscle with aging: Effects of exercise training. *Exercise and Sports Science Review, 21,* 65-102.

Shephard, R.J., & Åstrand, P.O. (1992). *Endurance in sport: The encyclopaedia of sports medicine* (Vol. 2). Oxford, UK: Blackwell Scientific.

Wilmore, J.H., & Costill, D.L. (1994). *Physiology of sport and exercise.* Champaign, IL: Human Kinetics.

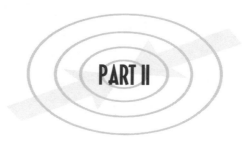

# PART II

# Physical Activity, Disease, and Disability

In part II, the link between physical activity and the major diseases experienced by modern-day men and women will be explored. The evidence for and against potential benefits of physical activity will be reviewed for such conditions as coronary heart disease, cancer, stroke, diabetes, arthritis, low back pain, asthma, infection, high blood cholesterol, high blood pressure, obesity, and stress. In general, although more research is needed for some disease areas, regular physical activity will be shown to have a strong effect in promoting health and preventing disease.

# Chapter 3

# CORONARY HEART DISEASE

Every man has two doctors, his right leg and his left.

(Ancient proverb)

The normal heart is a strong, muscular pump that, if given the chance, will beat nearly three billion times, pumping 42 million gallons of blood within one's lifetime. Unfortunately, many hearts have their work cut short by various diseases, most of which are caused by poor habits of living.

## Prevalence

Cardiovascular diseases, or CVD, are diseases of the heart and its blood vessels. Cardiovascular disease is not a single disorder; the term is a general name for more than 20 different diseases of the heart and its vessels. The American Heart Association has reminded us that although we have made tremendous progress in fighting CVD, these diseases have been the leading cause of death among Americans in every year but one (1918) since 1900. Four of every ten coffins contain victims of CVD.

Deaths, however, don't tell the whole story, because of the 255 million Americans, nearly one in four lives with some form of CVD. And one survey of 90,000 adults in the United States found that only 18 percent reported having no risk factors for heart disease. In other words, an alarming number of Americans either have CVD or are headed in that direction.

Cancer, according to most surveys, is the disease people fear the most. But CVD deserves more respect, maintains the National Center for Health Statistics. According to their most recent computations, if all forms of major CVD were eliminated, total life expectancy would rise by nearly 10 years. If all forms of cancer were abolished, the gain would be just 3 years.

# Pathology

Atherosclerosis, the buildup of fatty, plaque material in the inner layer of blood vessels, is the underlying factor in 85 percent of CVD. When the atherosclerotic plaque blocks one or more of the heart's coronary blood vessels, the diagnosis is coronary heart disease (CHD), the major form of CVD.

Often a blood clot forms in the narrowed coronary blood artery, blocking the blood flow to the part of the heart muscle supplied by that artery. This causes a heart attack or what clinicians call a myocardial infarction (MI). Each year, as many as 1,500,000 Americans have a heart attack, and about one-third of them will die.

The atherosclerosis can also block blood vessels in the brain (leading to a stroke) or legs (defined as peripheral artery disease). Stroke kills over 140,000 Americans each year, and is the third largest cause of death (this will be discussed further in chapter 5). Peripheral artery disease affects up to 20 percent of older people, and leads to pain in the legs brought on by walking (intermittent claudication). Patients with peripheral artery disease are able to walk only short distances before they must rest to relieve the pain in their legs brought on by poor circulation due to atherosclerosis.

Atherosclerosis begins with injury to the walls of the arteries. High blood cholesterol, high blood pressure, cigarette smoking, oxidized lipoproteins, and other factors all are capable of injuring the arteries. In response to the injury, monocytes, a type of white blood cell, are attracted, and crawl through spaces in the artery wall. They collect in the inner lining (called the intima) and are converted to macrophages, scavenger cells that engulf debris (see figure 3.1).

Cholesterol and triglycerides are carried through the bloodstream on lipoprotein particles. One type of lipoprotein, called the low-density lipoprotein (LDL), carries most of the blood's cholesterol. The LDL can be chemically modified by oxidation as a result of cigarette smoking or when the body's pool of vitamins A, E, and C (antioxidants found primarily in fruits and vegetables) is low because of poor diet. The oxidized LDL is engulfed by the macrophages, swelling the atherosclerotic plaque.

The oxidized LDL also injures the cells lining the blood vessel, attracting more monocytes from the bloodstream. The macrophages, as they engulf the LDL and other debris, release proteins that stimulate the production of collagen and other substances that make up the fibrous component of plaque. The net result of the atherosclerotic process is a progressive narrowing of the blood vessel opening, which ultimately leads to a heart attack, stroke, or peripheral artery disease.

## The Atherosclerotic Process

1. Artery wall is injured. High cholesterol, cigarette smoking, HBP, and other factors cause this.

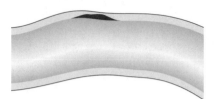

2. Monocytes collect at the injury site and become scavengers that collect debris. The scavengers are called macrophages.

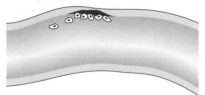

3. Low-density lipoproteins in the blood carry cholesterol and triglycerides. The macrophages engulf the LDL.

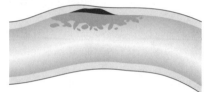

4. Macrophages release proteins that stimulate the production of collagen, further narrowing the artery.

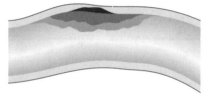

FIGURE 3.1    The atherosclerotic process.

Over the past quarter century, Americans have become increasingly health conscious and appreciative of the importance of disease prevention. As a result, death rates for heart disease have fallen significantly, and are half what they used to be during the middle part of the century.

Much has been written regarding the causes of this dramatic turnaround. There is no doubt that medical treatment of CHD has improved through use of new drugs and various surgical procedures. These include coronary artery bypass graft surgery, coronary angioplasty (using special catheters with small, inflatable balloons), laser angioplasty, coronary atherectomy (a special cutting device that grinds up plaque material), and coronary stents (metallic wire tubes used to keep the artery open).

Most experts feel, however, that the majority of the decline in CHD death rates is related to improvements in lifestyle by Americans, especially reductions in cigarette smoking and improvements in dietary quality and exercise habits. Lifestyle habits have a strong effect on CHD. In fact, up to 90 percent of CHD is thought to be preventable if only Americans would keep their risk factors under control through prudent living.

# EXERCISE-HEALTH CONNECTION

## What gives me the greatest risk of developing coronary heart disease?

Physical inactivity is a significant risk factor for CHD, even when other risk factors are accounted for. Taken together, studies suggest that inactivity in and of itself doubles the risk for CHD, an effect similar in magnitude to that of cigarette smoking or high blood pressure or cholesterol.

Risk factors are defined as personal habits or characteristics that medical research has shown to be associated with an increased risk of heart disease. Up until 1992, the American Heart Association did not include physical inactivity on its list of "major risk factors that can be changed," which included cigarette smoking, high blood pressure, and high blood cholesterol. Inactivity was listed along with obesity, stress, and diabetes among "contributing factors."

Heredity, gender (being a male), and increasing age have been listed for many years as "risk factors that cannot be changed." Table 3.1

TABLE 3.1

## Prevalence of Risk Factors for Heart Disease According to the American Heart Association

| Major risk factors that *can* be changed | % Americans with risk factor |
|---|---|
| 1. Cigarette smoking | 25% |
| 2. High blood pressure | 25% (>140/90 mmHg) |
| 3. High blood cholesterol | 20% (>240 mg/dl) |
| 4. Physical inactivity | 60% |
| **Major risk factors that *can't* be changed** | |
| 1. Heredity | —— |
| 2. Being male | —— |
| 3. Increasing age | 13% (over age 65) |
| **Other contributing factors** | |
| 1. Diabetes | 7% |
| 2. Obesity | 33% |
| 3. Stress | —— |

*Source:* American Heart Association.

outlines the current list of heart disease risk factors advanced by the American Heart Association, along with their current prevalence. Notice that among the risk factors listed, inactivity is by far the most prevalent, followed by obesity, cigarette smoking and high blood pressure, and then high blood cholesterol.

Why did the American Heart Association wait so long to include physical inactivity as a major risk factor for heart disease? The primary reason was that good research data to support this relationship was lacking until recently.

Most of the earlier studies showed that, compared to inactive people, physically active people had a lower risk for heart disease, but critics contended that other important factors were not controlled for in these studies. To state it another way, active people may be at lower risk, critics argued, because they also tend to eat more healthfully, are leaner, have lower blood pressure and cholesterol, are better educated, and may possess a better hereditary background than sedentary individuals.

For example, in one of the earliest studies, published in 1953, London busmen who sat and drove were found to be at higher risk for CHD than the conductors who moved through the double-decker buses collecting tickets. However, critics claimed that the drivers may have been at higher risk for CHD to begin with and may have "self-selected" themselves to an easier, sit-down type of job.

Dr. Ralph Paffenbarger of Stanford University has done more than any other researcher to silence the criticism and advance the cause of exercise as a valuable preventive measure. In 1970, Dr. Paffenbarger's research team published data showing that San Francisco longshoremen who did little physical labor on the job were at 60 percent greater risk for CHD death than colleagues engaging in physically demanding work.

In 1978, the first of several reports on college alumni was released, demonstrating that active alumni were at lower CHD risk than their inactive counterparts. In these studies, Dr. Paffenbarger carefully controlled for other CHD risk factors, showing that the sedentary lifestyle in and of itself was related to CHD.

Physical activity habits are difficult to measure, and assessment is largely based on information provided by the subjects. Cardiorespiratory fitness, however, is an objective measure and can be assessed rather easily.

Dr. Steven Blair of the Cooper Institute for Aerobics Research has been a leader in evaluating the relationship between fitness and CVD. He has used maximal treadmill testing (i.e., a steady increase in treadmill grade and speed to subject exhaustion) to measure cardiorespiratory fitness in a large group of men and women since 1970. Dr. Blair has found that a low level of fitness is a strong risk factor for CVD in both men and women. In fact, risk of CVD is up to eightfold greater for unfit groups as compared to their fit counterparts.

More research is needed with women. In one study from the University of Washington in Seattle, risk of heart attack among older women was decreased 50 percent with moderate amounts of exercise, equivalent to 30 to 45 minutes of walking, three times a week. Another study from the Brown University School of Medicine in Providence, Rhode Island, showed that the odds for CHD for sedentary women are more than doubled when compared to odds for their more active counterparts. These studies suggest that physical inactivity affects CHD risk to the same degree in men and women.

In 1987, a landmark review article was published by researchers from the Centers for Disease Control and Prevention (CDC). Of 43 studies reviewed, not one reported a greater risk for CHD among active participants. Two-thirds of the studies supported the finding that the physically active have less CHD than inactive people, and the studies following the best research design were the ones most likely to support this relationship.

In general, the studies taken together show that the risk for CHD among physically inactive people is twice that of people who are relatively active. This risk level is similar to that reported for high blood pressure, high blood cholesterol, and cigarette smoking. According to the CDC, regular physical activity should be promoted for CHD preven-

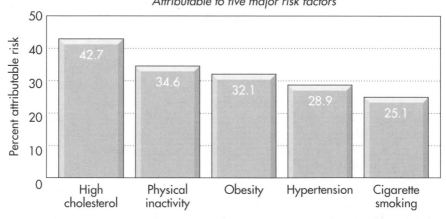

FIGURE 3.2  Physical inactivity ranks second in overall impact on CHD in America.

tion as vigorously as blood pressure control, dietary improvements to lower serum cholesterol and control weight, and smoking cessation.

It is the belief at the CDC that given the large proportion of Americans who do not exercise at appropriate levels (nearly 60 percent), the incidence of CHD that can actually be attributed to lack of regular physical activity is significant. Figure 3.2 summarizes the five leading risk factors for CHD in order of their overall impact on this disease in America. This rating takes into account two factors: the magnitude or strength of the risk factor's relationship to CHD, and the prevalence of the risk factor among Americans. Notice that inactivity ranks second to high blood cholesterol, with obesity, high blood pressure, and cigarette smoking ranked third, fourth, and fifth.

---

### How does exercise prevent coronary heart disease?

Fit people generally have other risk factors under good control. In addition, their hearts are larger and stronger, with an enhanced blood and oxygen supply, and with coronary arteries that can expand better and are larger and less stiff in older age.

---

Many experts feel that one of the most important reasons why active people have less CHD is that other risk factors are typically under control. For example, relatively few active people smoke cigarettes, are obese or diabetic, have high blood cholesterol, or experience high blood pressure. Active people have lower blood fats (i.e., triglycerides), have more high-density lipoprotein cholesterol (the "good" cholesterol), and generally report less anxiety and depression.

There is some controversy as to whether exercise or self-selection is responsible for these wonderful "side effects." In other words, does exercise attract people who are already healthy, or does it help people stop smoking, eat better, lose weight, lower blood pressure and cholesterol, manage stress, and avoid diabetes?

This question will be explored in greater detail in part II of this book. In general, although there is evidence in both directions, many experts feel that exercise does have a strong and direct effect in bringing many CHD risk factors under control.

Dr. Gary Fraser of the Center for Health Research at Loma Linda University suggests that the more good habits, the better, and that they are additive. For example, if by age 60 a male reports regular physical activity, he can expect to live an additional 5.7 years free of CHD beyond those reporting little activity. But if he has also avoided smoking, the benefit rises to 8.3 years. Low blood pressure and exercise together add up to 11.9 extra years free of CHD compared to the projection for inactive people with high blood pressure.

There are other important reasons why regular exercise is identified with lower CHD risk. Coronary arteries of endurance-trained individuals, for example, can expand more, are less stiff in older age, and are larger than those of unfit subjects. Even if some plaque material is present, the coronary arteries of fit people are large enough to diminish the risk of total closure leading to a heart attack.

Most heart attacks are triggered by clots. Although the issue is not yet settled, there is some evidence that exercise may decrease the potential for clot formation. In other words, with larger, more compliant coronary arteries, and a diminished aptitude to form clots, the active individual is at lower risk for a heart attack.

The heart muscle itself becomes bigger and stronger with regular exercise. Although still controversial, there is some indication that the fit heart develops extra blood vessels, enhancing blood and oxygen delivery.

One issue that nearly all experts agree on is that exercise must be a current and regular lifestyle habit in order for CHD risk to be lowered. In other words, people cannot "rest on their laurels" or "let the grass grow under their feet" and hope that the exercise habits of years gone by are sufficient for today.

In the College Alumni Studies, Dr. Paffenbarger noted that current physical activity habits were much more important when considering CHD risk than those from early adulthood. According to Dr. Paffenbarger, "Former college athletes who dropped their sports playing habits had higher death rates thereafter than their teammates who continued to exercise moderately vigorously into middle or later age. In contrast, college students who had avoided athletics in college but subsequently took up a more active lifestyle experienced the same low risk of mortality as alumni who had been moderately vigorous all along."

More recent results from the College Alumni Studies also support this concept. Risk of premature death from CHD was increased if physical activity was reduced below favorable levels, and risk was lowered if physical activity was increased. In fact, adopting a regular exercise program was found to be just as beneficial in lowering CHD risk as were quitting smoking and avoiding obesity and high blood pressure.

These results are similar to those of Dr. Blair, who showed that individuals maintaining or improving fitness over a five-year span were less likely to die from CVD than those who stayed unfit. Men in the Aerobics Center Longitudinal Study who improved their fitness during the five-year study had a 64 percent reduction in risk of death, greater than for any of the other risk factors.

---

### How much exercise is necessary to lower my risk of heart disease?

About 30 minutes of moderate-intensity physical activity a day is sufficient, with risk lowered even further when greater amounts of more vigorous exercise are engaged in.

---

There has been some debate as to the volume and intensity of exercise essential for lowering CHD risk. Some studies have indicated that regular and vigorous exercise is necessary, while others suggest that exercise of moderate duration and intensity is sufficient to reduce CHD risk.

There is increasing consensus that while moderate exercise is a "sufficient threshold" for lowering CHD risk, additional benefit is gained when people are willing to exercise more vigorously for longer periods of time. However, the relationship does not appear to be linear. The greatest CHD risk benefit occurs when sedentary people adopt moderate physical activity habits, with some additional protection gained as the duration and intensity of exercise are raised to a higher level.

Dr. Blair has emphasized that as little as two miles of brisk walking on most days of the week would result in the moderate level of fitness shown in the Aerobics Center Longitudinal Study to be protective. Other studies suggest a level of activity just a bit higher, the equivalent of two to three miles of brisk walking each day of the week.

An expert panel convened by the National Institutes of Health concluded that "activity that reduces CVD risk factors and confers many other health benefits does not require a structured or vigorous exercise program. The majority of benefits of physical activity can be gained by performing moderate-intensity activities. . . . We recommend that all children and adults should set a long-term goal to accumulate at least 30 minutes or more of moderate-intensity physical activity on most, or preferably all, days of the week."

Some researchers, however, urge that people should not be mistaken that a casual approach to fitness is sufficient. Dr. Timo Lakka of the University of Kuopio in Finland did a five-year study of 1,453 middle-aged men who were initially free of CHD. He classified subjects based on the frequency and intensity of their leisure-time physical activity. Men who engaged in moderate-to-strenuous activity for at least 2.2 hours per week had a risk of heart attack that was less than half the risk of the least active men. Only moderate-to-strenuous aerobic activities such as brisk walking, jogging, bicycling, or cross-country skiing were shown to confer protection. Nonconditioning activities such as slow walking, fishing, easy yard work or gardening, hunting, or picking berries did not lower CHD risk.

---

### If I have atherosclerosis, will exercise cure it?

Studies have shown that intensive drug and/or lifestyle therapy (including exercise as one of several components) leading to marked improvements in blood lipids generally result in more regression or less progression of plaque buildup than among "usual care" controls.

---

Preventing atherosclerosis from forming in the first place is the principal strategy each individual should embrace. However, for those who have had a heart attack or are at high CHD risk, can the atherosclerosis already accumulated be reversed? Can dietary changes, exercise, weight loss, smoking cessation, stress management, and/or drug therapy both prevent and reverse the buildup of plaque?

Since early in this century, regression of atherosclerosis has been demonstrated in many different types of animals, including rabbits, chickens, dogs, pigeons, pigs, and monkeys. In the typical animal experiment, atherosclerosis is promoted by a diet high in fat and cholesterol, followed by a near-vegetarian "regression" diet that leads to a reduction in plaque size.

In the 1970s, studies with rhesus monkeys showed that a high-fat, cholesterol-rich diet for just 17 months clogged the coronaries 60 percent with plaque material, while a low-fat, no-cholesterol diet for 40 months reversed it by two-thirds. Other animal studies showed that almost total reversal could be achieved if the atherosclerosis was relatively new.

In 1981, a landmark study was published showing that aerobic exercise has an important role in retarding the growth of atherosclerosis in monkeys. Monkeys were fed a high-fat, high-cholesterol diet. When compared to sedentary monkeys, those that were exercised had larger coronary arteries with less obstruction. Studies with pigs also produced the same result, confirming that exercise was an important factor in countering the buildup of plaque.

Studies with humans have been difficult to achieve because indirect measures of coronary blockage are complex. In other words, because humans cannot be sacrificed and autopsied like animals, less precise measures such as coronary arteriography and positron emission tomography (PET), have placed limits on what can be achieved with human subjects.

Nonetheless, during the last two decades as technology has improved, studies have shown that intensive drug and diet therapy leading to marked improvements in blood fats retards the progression of coronary atherosclerosis, promotes regression, and thus decreases the incidence of coronary events.

In one review of 12 of the best studies, it was determined that diet and/or lifestyle interventions with heart disease patients over an average of 3.3 years had notable effects on atherosclerosis. Among control patients not on the intervention regimen, 52 percent experienced progression, 9 percent regression, and 39 percent no change, in comparison to 24, 27, and 49 percent, respectively, among patients on treatment. More impressively, patients in treatment experienced 50 percent fewer cardiovascular events (e.g., heart attacks, death).

Can lifestyle treatment alone without drug therapy produce similar results? In one study (called the Lifestyle Heart Trial) headed by Dr. Dean Ornish of the University of California at San Francisco, heart disease patients were placed on an extremely low-fat vegetarian diet (7 percent calories as fat) and given stress management and moderate exercise. The treatment subjects lost an average of 22 pounds and lowered their cholesterol from 227 to 172 mg/dl (24 percent reduction); 82 percent of them experienced regression compared to 42 percent of controls. Patients in the treatment group also reported a 91 percent reduction in the frequency of angina pain compared to a 165 percent rise among controls.

These patients were followed for over five years, and those adhering to the strict lifestyle standards continued to experience impressive benefits relative to controls. A 39-month study of 90 heart disease patients in England has confirmed the value of diet therapy, concluding that diet alone can retard the overall progression and increase overall regression of coronary artery disease.

In Germany, researchers have studied the effects of exercise in regression of coronary atherosclerosis. Heart disease patients were assigned to an intervention group that exercised several hours a week or a control group receiving usual care. After one year, among patients exercising, regression of coronary artery disease was measured in 28 percent, progression in 10 percent, and no change in 62 percent, while among controls, the results were 6, 45, and 49 percent, respectively. The researchers concluded that regression of coronary artery disease is likely among patients who expend 2,200 calories per week in exercise (about five to six hours weekly).

This same German research team also showed that in patients combining exercise with a low-fat diet, coronary artery disease progressed at a slower pace than in a control group on usual care. The challenge, as these investigators have noted, is getting patients to adhere to the improved lifestyle over long time periods.

---

### If I have coronary heart disease, will exercise cure it?

Yes, especially when combined with other lifestyle changes such as smoking cessation, weight control, and dietary improvement. When all studies are evaluated together, total and CVD mortality are reduced 20 to 25 percent for patients in cardiac rehabilitation programs (of which exercise is usually the key component) compared to those not participating.

---

Each year, about 1.5 million Americans have a heart attack. Although one-third die soon afterward, the majority live to face an uncertain future. People who survive the acute stage of a heart attack have a chance of illness and death two to nine times higher than the general population. During the first year after having a heart attack, 27 percent of men and 44 percent of women will die. Over 11 million Americans alive today have a history of heart attack, angina pectoris (chest pain), or both.

Cardiovascular operations and procedures to treat heart disease are a growing industry. Total vascular and cardiac surgeries now number over 4.4 million per year, including diagnostic cardiac catheterizations, coronary artery bypass graft surgery, percutaneous transluminal coronary angioplasty, open heart surgery, heart transplants, and pacemaker insertions.

Cardiac rehabilitation programs were first developed in the 1950s in response to the growing epidemic of heart disease. Participants include people who have CHD, those who have had a heart attack, and surgery patients. Many programs admit people who have multiple CHD risk factors but have not yet been diagnosed with CVD. The goal is to prepare cardiac patients to return to productive, active, and satisfying lives with a reduced risk of recurring health problems.

The emphasis in cardiac rehabilitation programs is usually on lifestyle change, optimization of drug therapy, vocational counseling, and group and family therapy. Regarding lifestyle change, exercise is considered the cornerstone, but weight control, smoking cessation, and dietary therapy are also essential.

During the early days of cardiac rehabilitation, it was common practice to have the heart attack patient stay in bed a minimum of two to three weeks. As research began to demonstrate the importance of early and progressive physical activity, a four-phase plan was developed that is now standard in most programs. Patients with no complications are expected to progress from phase I through phase III within one year after an acute cardiac event. Phase IV is designed for lifelong exercise participation. Phase I is easy walking and bed exercises during the first 5 to 14 days while the patient is in the coronary care unit of the hospital. Phase II is an outpatient program lasting one to three months, with the patient exercising aerobically in the hospital or clinic under careful supervision. Phase III, lasting 6 to 12 months, is a supervised aerobic exercise program in a community setting.

Exercise programs for cardiac patients should be highly individualized and should involve an initial slow, gradual progression of the exercise duration and intensity. Aerobic activities should be emphasized, with a minimum frequency of three days per week, 20-40 minutes each session, at a moderate, comfortable intensity. Some resistance exercise, but at a low intensity, is recommended to help build up weakened muscles.

Unfortunately, only 15 percent of eligible cardiac patients actually participate in cardiac rehabilitation programs. For a variety of reasons, these programs are not feasible or desirable for the vast majority of patients. One problem is that phases II and III involve medical supervision at a designated site (hospital, clinic, or fitness center). This presents time and transportation obstacles for many patients. Home-based programs, an attractive alternative, provide a convenient setting and can also involve the support of family members.

Several pertinent questions have been raised regarding cardiac rehabilitation programs. Do they increase the aerobic fitness of cardiac patients? Do they lengthen life and lower the risk of new cardiac events? Are they safe?

Many studies have clearly shown that cardiac patients who exercise regularly improve their aerobic fitness. $VO_2$max increases by an average of 20 percent, according to most studies, and anginal symptoms often disappear or take longer to develop during a given exercise load.

Researchers have been unable to provide a clear picture as to whether or not exercise by cardiac patients leads to longer life or fewer subsequent heart attacks. Two review articles have shown that when all studies are gathered together, total and CVD mortality are reduced 20-

25 percent for patients in cardiac rehabilitation programs as compared to those not participating. However, the programs involved more than just exercise training, so it is difficult to quantify the role of exercise alone.

Comprehensive cardiac rehabilitation programs that include exercise, diet, and other health behavior changes do help patients keep their CHD risk factors under tighter control. Perhaps more importantly, studies show that patients in cardiac rehabilitation programs report an improved quality of life.

Cardiac rehabilitation programs are safe. The estimated incidence of heart attack in supervised cardiac rehabilitation programs is only 1 per 294,000 patient-hours, and for death, 1 per 784,000 patient-hours. Over 80 percent of patients who were reported to have experienced a cardiac arrest while in a cardiac rehabilitation program have been successfully resuscitated with prompt defibrillation.

The American College of Sports Medicine concludes that "most patients with coronary artery disease should engage in individually designed exercise programs to achieve optimal physical and emotional health. . . . Appropriate exercise programs for patients with coronary artery disease have multiple documented benefits, which can be achieved with a high level of safety."

# PRECAUTIONS: BALANCING BENEFITS AND RISKS

For some individuals, both young and old, exercise can actually cause a heart attack. However, with the appropriate precautions, most of these deaths can be prevented.

---

### Is there a risk of dying of a heart attack during exercise?

Yes, a small risk does exist. But most people over age 30 who have a heart attack during or after vigorous exercise are at high risk for CHD and then exercise too hard for their fitness level, triggering the final heart attack event. For younger people, the cause is usually heart or blood vessel birth defects. If an individual is at low risk for heart disease, has not experienced any symptoms, and exercises moderately, risk is extremely low, and overall, heart disease risk should be lowered because of the regular exercise program.

---

There's probably not a single fitness enthusiast in America who hasn't read the reports of famous athletes dying on basketball courts, runners found dead with their running shoes on, executives discovered slumped over their treadmills, or middle-aged fathers unearthed alongside their snow shovels. Examples include author and marathon runner Jim Fixx, basketball stars Reggie Lewis, "Pistol Pete" Maravich, and Hank Gathers, and MCI chairman Bill McGowan. During the "blizzard of the century" in 1993, scores of people along the eastern seaboard died of sudden heart attack while shoveling snow from their driveways.

For most people, regular physical activity can be expected to cut their risk of CHD in half. For others, this protective weapon may reveal itself as a two-edged sword.

Whether exercise is beneficial or hazardous to the heart appears to depend on who the person is. In one study of 100 athletes who died young (average age 18), suddenly, and in their prime while exercising, 90 of them had heart or blood vessel birth defects. Most common was hypertrophic cardiomyopathy, a thickening of the heart's main pumping muscle.

In other words, when a young athlete dies during or shortly after exercise, it is most often due to a defect in the structure of the heart or blood vessel that was present at birth. In fact, congenital CVD is now the major cause of athletic death in high school and college. Despite the relative rarity of these types of deaths and the cost of testing, there are renewed calls by many experts for examinations of young athletes prior to sport participation. There are some exceptions to the rule that young athletes who die suddenly tend to have congenital defects in their hearts and blood vessels. For example, in 1995, the 28-year-old Russian ice skater Sergei Grinkov died of a heart attack during practice. An autopsy showed that two coronary arteries in Grinkov's heart were blocked. There was a history of heart disease in his family, including his father, who had died in his mid-40s.

For most individuals over age 30 who die during or shortly after exercise, the cause is from a narrowing of the coronary blood vessels of the heart from atherosclerosis. It appears that when people with these narrowed coronary blood vessels exert themselves heavily during exercise, the increase in heart rate and blood pressure may cause a disruption of the deposits, setting in motion a chain of events that causes a complete blockage and heart attack.

To state it another way, middle-aged and older adults who die during exercise tend to be people who already have some heart disease. They are at high risk to begin with, and then the vigorous exercise triggers the final heart attack event.

Researchers from Harvard studied the heart attack episodes of 1,228 men and women and found that the risk was 5.9 times higher after heavy exertion versus lighter or no exertion. Heavy physical exertion was especially risky for people who were habitually inactive. In other words, people who usually exercised very little, and then went out and exercised vigorously (e.g., shoveled snow), were much more likely to have experienced a heart attack than those who were accustomed to exercise.

These researchers concluded that every year in the United States, 75,000 Americans experience a heart attack during or after vigorous exercise, and that these individuals tend to be sedentary and at high risk for heart attack to begin with. Another study from Germany has also concluded that "a period of strenuous physical activity is associated with a temporary increase in the risk of having a myocardial infarction, particularly among patients who exercise infrequently."

In one study of 36 marathon runners who had died suddenly or had a heart attack, researchers found that in most of the cases a strong family history of heart disease, high blood cholesterol, or early warning symptoms (e.g., chest pain) were present. Most of the runners had symptoms of heart disease, but denied they had them, and continued training and racing until they finally had a heart attack or died.

It is important to understand it is rare for a heart attack to occur during exercise, despite the media reports. Most researchers have found that in a given year, fewer than 10 out of 100,000 men will have a heart attack during exercise. These people tend to be men who were sedentary and already had heart disease or were at high risk for it, and then exercised too hard for their fitness level.

People at high risk for heart disease should avoid heavy exertion until being cleared by their physicians after taking a maximal treadmill electrocardiogram (EKG) test. According to the American College of Sports Medicine, "The incidence of cardiovascular problems during physical activity is reduced by nearly 50% when individuals are first screened and those identified with risk factors or disease are diverted to other professionally established activity programs." Even after clearance, intense exercise should be avoided until fitness has been gradually improved and heart disease risk factors have been brought under control.

Certain physical activities that seem benign should be approached cautiously by those at high CHD risk. For example, heavy snow shoveling has been shown to cause marked increases in heart rate and blood pressure, which may explain the common press reports of excess cardiac deaths after heavy snowfalls. Figure 3.3 outlines recommendations for intensity of exercise using the rating of perceived exertion scale.

| | Exercise CHD Risk vs. Benefit |
|---|---|
| 6 | **Using the Rating of Perceived Exertion** |
| 7 Very, very light | |
| 8 | LIGHT EXERCISE |
| 9 Very light | Some CHD benefits, but |
| 10 | minimal fitness improvement |
| 11 Fairly light | |
| 12 | MODERATE EXERCISE |
| 13 Somewhat hard | Both CHD and fitness |
| 14 | benefits with minimal risk |
| 15 Hard | |
| 16 | INTENSE EXERCISE |
| 17 Very hard | For those who desire high |
| 18 Very, very hard | fitness. Can precipitate |
| 19 Maximal | heart attack in high risk. |

**FIGURE 3.3**    Risk of heart attack during exercise rises with increase in exercise intensity. Borg, G. An introduction to Borg's RPE scale. Ithaca, NY: Movement Publications, 1985.

# REFERENCES

American College of Sports Medicine. (1994). Exercise for patients with coronary artery disease. *Medicine and Science in Sports and Exercise, 26*, i-v.

American Heart Association. (1996). *Heart and stroke facts: 1997 statistical update*. Dallas: American Heart Association.

Amsterdam, E.A., Hyson, D., & Kappagoda, C.T. (1994). Nonpharmacologic therapy for coronary artery atherosclerosis: Results of primary and secondary prevention trials. *American Heart Journal, 128*, 134-1352.

Blair, S.N., Kohl, H.W., Barlow, C.E., Paffenbarger, R.S., Gibbons, L.W., & Macera, C.A. (1995). Changes in physical fitness and all-cause mortality: A prospective study of healthy and unhealthy men. *Journal of the American Medical Association, 273*, 1093-1098.

Fletcher, G.F., Blair, S.N., Blumenthal, J., et al. (1992). Benefits and recommendations for physical activity programs for all Americans. A statement for health professionals by the committee on exercise and cardiac rehabilitation of the Council on Clinical Cardiology, American Heart Association. *Circulation, 86*, 340-343.

Fraser, G.E., Lindstead, K.D., & Beeson, W.L. (1995). Effect of risk factor values on lifetime risk of and age at first coronary event: The Adventist Health Study. *American Journal of Epidemiology, 142*, 746-758.

Lakka, T.A., Venäläinen, J.M., Rauramaa, R., Salonen, R., Tuomilehto, J., & Salonen, J.T. (1994). Relation of leisure-time physical activity and cardiorespiratory fitness to the risk of acute myocardial infarction in men. *New England Journal of Medicine, 330*, 1549-1554.

Lemaitre, R.N., Heckbert, S.R., Psaty, B.M., & Siscovick, D.S. (1995). Leisure-time physical activity and the risk of nonfatal myocardial infarction in postmenopausal women. *Archives of Internal Medicine, 155,* 2302-2308.

Margolis, S., & Goldschmidt-Clermont, P.J. (1995). *The Johns Hopkins white papers, coronary heart disease.* Baltimore: The Johns Hopkins Medical Institutions.

Nieman, D.C. (1995). *Fitness and sports medicine: A health-related approach.* Mountain View, CA: Mayfield Publishing.

NIH Consensus Development Panel on Physical Activity and Cardiovascular Health. (1996). Physical activity and cardiovascular health. *Journal of the American Medical Association, 276,* 241-246.

Paffenbarger, R.S., Kampert, J.B., Lee, I-M., Hyde, R.T., Leung, R.W., & Wing, A.L. (1994). Changes in physical activity and other lifeway patterns influencing longevity. *Medicine and Science in Sports and Exercise, 26,* 857-865.

Powell, K.E., Thompson, P.D., Caspersen, C.J., & Kendrick, J.S. (1987). Physical activity and the incidence of coronary heart disease. *Annual Review of Public Health, 8,* 253-287.

U.S. Department of Health and Human Services. (1996). *Physical activity and health: A report of the Surgeon General.* Atlanta: U.S. Department of Health and Human Services, Centers for Disease Control and Prevention, National Center for Chronic Disease Prevention and Health Promotion.

Willich, S.N., Lewis, M., Löwel, H., Arntz, H.-R., Schubert, F., and Schröder, R. (1993). Physical exertion as a trigger of acute myocardial infarction. *New England Journal of Medicine, 329,* 1684-1690.

# Chapter 4

# CANCER

*If everything known about the prevention of cancer was applied,*
*up to two-thirds of cancers would not occur.*

**American Cancer Society**

Although heart disease is America's leading killer, cancer is the disease feared by most mortals. And for good reason. According to Dr. Debra Davis, the Assistant Secretary for Health, Department of Health and Human Services, "The bad news is that in all age groups cancer incidence is increasing . . . and that few new effective treatments have been devised for the most common cancers."

## Prevalence

Since the mid-1960s, the percentage of deaths from heart disease has fallen fairly consistently, from 39 percent of all deaths at that time to 32 percent in the mid-1990s. Meanwhile, the percentage of total deaths attributed to cancer rose from 16 to 24 percent. Soon after the turn of the next century, cancer is expected to emerge as America's leading cause of death.

The National Cancer Institute has estimated that the lifetime risk of developing cancer is a staggering 45 percent for men and 39 percent for women. Among men, 23 percent will die of cancer, whereas 20 percent of women will succumb.

More than 1.36 million Americans are diagnosed with cancer each year (not including the more than 800,000 cases of skin cancer). Each year, over one-half million Americans die of cancer, about 1,500 each day. The leading cancer killer for both men and women is lung cancer, followed by prostate or breast cancer, and colorectal cancer.

These are alarming statistics, and the primary solution, according to Dr. Lawrence Garfinkel of the American Cancer Society, is "more education concerning the importance of curtailing and/or preventing those lifestyle risk factors over which a person has control."

## Pathology

There are many types of cancers, but they can all be characterized by uncontrolled growth and spread of abnormal cells. If the spread is not controlled, it can result in death as vital passageways are blocked and the body's oxygen and nutrient supply is diverted to support the rapidly growing cancer.

Humans are made up of approximately 60 trillion cells. Each cell contains DNA, the blueprint for making enzymes that drive unique chemical reactions. Dr. Bruce Ames, a professor of molecular and cellular biology at the University of California at Berkeley, has estimated that the DNA in each cell receives a "hit" once every 10 seconds from damaging molecules.

Most of the DNA injury comes from a class of chemicals known as oxidants, byproducts of the normal process by which cells turn food into energy. Although much of the damage is repaired, over a lifetime the unrepaired damage accumulates. In Ames's view, both the process of aging and the incidence of cancer can be attributed in large part to the accumulation of damage to DNA. Not only will alteration of the DNA affect the cell in which it occurs, but when that cell divides, the defective blueprint will be passed on to all the descendants of that cell.

Normally the cells that make up the body reproduce and divide in an orderly manner, so that old cells are replaced and cell injuries repaired. Supported by certain environmental (e.g., oxidants and other chemicals, radiation, and viruses) and internal (e.g., hormones, immune conditions, and inherited mutations) factors, some cells undergo abnormal changes and begin the process (often taking longer than 10 years) toward becoming a cancer cell.

These abnormal cells may grow into masses of tissue called tumors, some of which are cancerous and others benign. The danger of malignant cancer cells is that they invade neighboring or distant organs or tissues. If left untreated, the cancer can spread throughout the body, quickly leading to advanced cancer and death.

## Prognosis

In the early 1900s, few cancer patients had much hope of long-term survival. In the 1930s, fewer than 1 person in 5 was alive five years after treatment. Now, 4 of 10 patients who get cancer live five or more years after diagnosis. With regular screening and self-exams, cancer can often be detected early, greatly enhancing the success of treatment.

## Prevention

Throughout the world, cancer death rates vary widely, with industrial countries leading the list. Researchers have carefully demonstrated that when migrants adopt westernized lifestyles, certain types of cancers, especially colon, breast, and prostate, increase. About 35 percent of cancer is now attributed to dietary factors, and 30 percent to cigarette smoking.

The American Cancer Society has urged that Americans avoid all tobacco use and consume low-fat, high-fiber diets containing plenty of whole grains, fruits, and vegetables to reduce cancer risk. Numerous studies have shown that daily consumption of vegetables and fruits is associated with a reduced risk of lung, prostate, bladder, esophagus, and stomach cancers. Vegetables and fruits contain antioxidant vitamins (A, C, E, and the provitamin beta-carotene), minerals, fiber, and nonnutritive substances that together reduce cancer risk. Plant foods, especially whole-grain cereals, contain dietary fiber that helps protect against colon cancer.

Regular physical activity was finally added in 1996 to the list of preventive measures advocated by the American Cancer Society. The American Heart Association also took a long time (until the early 1990s) to identify physical inactivity as a risk factor for heart disease. The link between chronic disease and inactivity is a difficult one to establish because the relationship is complex, with many other lifestyle factors (difficult to measure) affecting the process.

Evidence is mounting that inactivity does contribute to the development of cancer, and this chapter will summarize important findings. Although the epidemic of heart disease during the mid-20th century diverted the attention of researchers, the fact that cancer deaths are increasing has revitalized the nation's determination to wage war against cancer.

More and more exercise scientists are joining the fray, and physical inactivity should soon emerge as a cancer risk factor that parallels its impact on heart disease. As emphasized by one of the world's leading researchers in this area, Dr. I-Min Lee of the Harvard School of Public Health, "Our findings now suggest that increased physical activity may reduce the risk of certain types of cancer, especially colon cancer."

# INACTIVITY AS A RISK FACTOR FOR CANCER

Fred Lebow came to the United States in 1951, a Romanian-born Jew with grand vision, ambition, and a gift for hard work and pragmatism. He also loved to run, and in 1972 took over as president of the New York Runners Club. Lebow founded and organized several major road races including the New York City Marathon, now one of the world's largest. A marathon runner himself, he competed in 69 marathon race events, training year-round to keep in shape.

Lebow was shocked and surprised when he was diagnosed with brain cancer in February of 1990. But in keeping with his irrepressible will, even as he underwent chemotherapy he continued to run, first on the roof of the hospital and then back out on the roads and paths of Central Park. In 1992, he and an old friend, nine-time New York City Marathon winner Grete Waitz of Norway, ran the entire 26.2-mile course, cheered on every step of the way by admiring citizens of the Big Apple.

Just before the 1994 New York City Marathon, runners throughout the world were saddened to hear that Fred Lebow had died at age 62 after a second bout with brain cancer. Lebow's fight against cancer was well known, and has raised two important questions in the minds of many runners and fitness enthusiasts: (1) Why did Fred Lebow get cancer in the first place—isn't exercise supposed to lower the risk? and (2) Should he have cut back on his training after being diagnosed with cancer? Can too much exercise be harmful to the cancer patient? And on the other hand, can moderate amounts be beneficial?

---

*Can I avoid getting cancer if I exercise every day?*
*Is exercise more effective at preventing some*
*cancers than others?*

Yes, especially for colon, breast, and prostate cancer and perhaps some other female reproductive cancers (e.g., uterine).

---

The idea that increased physical exercise may be of benefit in preventing cancer is not a new one. More than 70 years ago, researchers in Australia observed that primitive tribes who labored continuously for food had lower rates of cancer than people from more civilized societies. Other scientists and physicians observed early in this century that most cancer patients had led relatively sedentary lives, and that men who had worked hard all their lives had less cancer than those who tended to sit during their day of work.

These fascinating findings lay dormant until just the past 10 to 15 years, when researchers throughout the world took up the question anew. Since then, many studies have bolstered the evidence of an exercise-cancer connection. Active animals, former athletes, people employed in active occupations, and those who exercise after work hours have been compared to their sedentary counterparts. In general, depending on the type of cancer site investigated, they have been found to have a lower risk of cancer. The Institute for Aerobics Research in Dallas, Texas, for example, recently showed that over an eight-year period, physically unfit men had four times the overall cancer death rate of the most fit men, with an even wider spread found among the women.

Several researchers have injected animals with certain types of cancer-causing chemicals, divided them into exercise and nonexercise groups, and then measured the size and time of cancer appearance. Results consistently show that exercise tends to retard cancer growth at several different sites. Dr. Laurie Hoffman-Goetz of the University of Waterloo in Ontario, Canada, for example, exercised mice for nine weeks and found that they were better able to clear certain types of cancer cells from their bodies than physically inactive mice.

Although Dr. Hoffman-Goetz emphasizes that more research is needed, she feels that exercise training improves the cancer-fighting proficiency of natural killer cells. These are an important type of white blood cell in the body that provides natural immunity against some forms of cancer. Dr. Mark Davis of the School of Public Health, University of South Carolina, has shown that after each exercise bout, macrophages (another important white blood cell) are more active than normal for several hours in destroying cancer cells in mice.

Large groups of people have been followed for extended periods of time to see if those who exercise regularly have less cancer than those who lead an inactive lifestyle. The most impressive results have shown a protective effect of exercise against three common cancer killers: colon, breast, and prostate cancer. Although more research is needed, most experts feel that it is unlikely that physical activity has a strong influence on other cancers at sites such as the lung, pancreas, bladder, stomach, or oral cavity.

Most experts feel that cancer prevention can be added to the long list of benefits identified with regular, daily, moderate exercise. Although it is not clear how much exercise it takes to help prevent cancer, researchers agree that the single most important factor is consistency.

Since cancer is a disease that can take years or even decades to develop, exercise should be a regular part of the daily routine to ensure that it has a measurable and long-term effect on cancer prevention.

---

*You've said that regular exercise lowers the risk of getting colon, prostate, breast, and female reproductive cancers. How?*

Among all cancer sites, exercise is most beneficial in preventing cancer of the colon. Researchers think that's because exercise may help the contents of the colon move along faster, keep people lean, and lower blood insulin levels; all these effects lower colon cancer risk.

---

Increasing evidence suggests that women who engage in vigorous exercise from early in life may gain some protection against breast cancer, and that vigorous exercise may help decrease exposure of the breast to female hormones, diminishing the potential for cancer cells to develop. There is limited but consistent evidence that sedentary compared to physically active women are at higher risk for uterine cancer.

More research is needed to determine whether physical activity reduces the risk of prostate cancer. Higher levels of testosterone may contribute to the development of prostate cancer, and it seems that highly active men may expose their prostate to less testosterone.

## Colon Cancer

Each year, more than 140,000 new cases and 55,000 deaths occur in the United States from colon and rectum cancer. Early detection is critical; the American Cancer Society recommends digital rectal exams starting at age 40, and stool blood testing and proctosigmoidoscopy (insertion of a hollow, lighted tube to inspect the rectum and lower colon) starting at age 50.

Major risk factors include family history and a high-fat, low-fiber diet. Colon and rectum cancer varies markedly from one nation to another. For example, it is rare in southwest Asia and equatorial Africa, but common throughout northwestern Europe, the United States, and Canada.

Studies of migrants have shown the importance of environmental and lifestyle factors in colon cancer. For example, the death rate for colorectal cancer in Japanese immigrants to the United States is three to four times greater than that of Japanese in Japan. Puerto Ricans in New York City have more colon cancer than those remaining in Puerto Rico.

Although the precise causes of colon cancer remain unclear, a diet high in red meat or animal fat and low in fruits and vegetables appears to increase the risk for colorectal cancer. It has been estimated that an increase in dietary fiber intake of 13 grams per day would reduce colorectal cancer risk by 31 percent. Currently, the average American consumes 12-18 grams of dietary fiber a day, below the 20-30 grams recommended by the National Cancer Institute. In one study of nearly 90,000 nurses, intake of animal fat and meat was strongly associated with the risk of colon cancer. Vegetarians, who eat more fiber and less animal fat than meat-eaters, have a much lower risk of colon cancer.

High-fat diets increase bile acid production, which can be transformed by colonic bacteria into cancer-causing chemicals. Dietary fiber binds bile acids, increases stool bulk, speeds up the movement of the fecal mass through the colon, and thereby reduces the exposure of bile acid products to the colon wall.

About 35 studies have been published that looked at both occupational and leisure-time physical activity in relation to colon cancer. Three-fourths of these studies showed that physically active compared to inactive people have less colon cancer. The protective effect of physical activity against colon cancer has been seen in several countries, including China, Sweden, Japan, and the United States. A frequent finding has been that people who tend to sit for the majority of their workday or remain inactive in their leisure time have a 30 to 100 percent greater risk of contracting colon cancer. For example, researchers at the University of Southern California studied nearly 3,000 men with colon cancer and compared them with the rest of the male population of Los Angeles County. The men who worked at sedentary jobs were found to have a 60 percent greater colon cancer risk.

Dr. Matthew Longnecker studied 163 colon cancer patients and 703 controls, and found that two hours per week or more of vigorous leisure-time physical activity (e.g., running, bicycling, lap swimming, racquet sports, calisthenics, and rowing) lowered the risk for colon cancer by 40 percent. Dr. Longnecker concluded, "The consistency of the findings that physical activity is inversely related to risk of colon cancer is greater than is the evidence that dietary factors affect risk, and suggests physical activity may be an especially effective public health intervention."

Researchers at Harvard University studied 48,000 male health professionals and showed that colon cancer risk was decreased 50 percent in the most physically active men compared to their sedentary peers (see figure 4.1). The protective effect was most evident in men who exercised

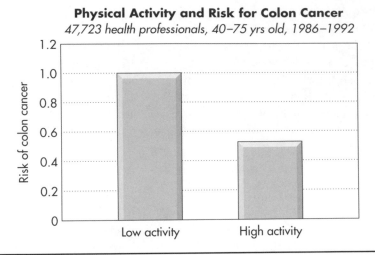

**Physical Activity and Risk for Colon Cancer**
*47,723 health professionals, 40–75 yrs old, 1986–1992*

FIGURE 4.1   Active individuals greatly reduce their risk of developing colon cancer.

on average about one to two hours a day. Men who were both physically inactive and obese had a colon cancer risk that was nearly five times higher than that of their active and lean counterparts.

One theory is that each exercise bout stimulates muscle movement (peristalsis) of the large intestine. This shortens the time that various cancer-causing chemicals in the fecal matter stay in contact with the cells that line the colon. In other words, exercise has an effect on the colon similar to the effect of dietary fiber.

It is well known that those who exercise suffer less often from constipation than do the sedentary. In one large national survey, people were asked, "Do you have trouble with your bowels that makes you constipated?" Among middle-aged adults, twice as many of those reporting "little exercise" had trouble with constipation as compared to highly active people.

Other theories have been proposed. In animal studies, when caloric intake is slightly below body needs, cancer risk is lowered. In fact, this is one of the strongest variables controlling cancer in animals. Regular exercise seems to help some people control their dietary intake. As a result, active people tend to be less obese, which is important because obesity in and of itself promotes several different types of cancer, including colon cancer. Both obesity and physical inactivity promote higher blood levels of insulin, a hormone that increases the growth rate of cells lining the colon and hence their likelihood of turning cancerous.

Active people may also eat more dietary fiber, enhancing their protection against colon cancer. For example, in the study from Harvard

University reviewed earlier in this chapter, highly active men ate 29 grams of dietary fiber a day, more than double the intake (12 grams) of the inactive men. It should be noted, however, than even after controlling for dietary fiber intake, physical activity still in and of itself lowered colon cancer risk.

## Breast Cancer

Of the various female reproductive cancers (breast, uterus, and ovary), breast cancer has been the most commonly studied. American women have a one in eight likelihood of developing breast cancer within their lifetimes. Each year, an estimated 182,000 women develop breast cancer and 46,000 die of it. Early detection is critical, and the American Cancer Society recommends a screening mammogram starting at age 40, with clinical breast exams starting at age 20.

The risk of breast cancer increases with age. Between 40 and 50 percent of breast cancer cases can be explained by four well-established risk factors: never had children, late age at first live birth, high education and socioeconomic status, and family history of breast cancer. Early age at menarche, late age at menopause, and obesity are also important risk factors. Certain types of breast cancer are strongly inheritable, and studies with identical twins have shown that if one twin acquires breast cancer, the risk for the other twin is six times greater than normal and usually occurs in the same breast (right or left).

The development of breast cancer is related to female hormones, since it occurs many times more frequently in women than in men and can be prevented by removal of the ovaries early in life. Any factor that lessens reproductive hormone exposure for a woman (e.g., later menarche or early menopause) reduces breast cancer risk.

As with colon cancer, breast cancer death rates vary widely between nations, and the difference is not explained by genetics. Breast cancer rates are four to seven times higher in the United States than in Asia. When women migrate from geographic areas with low rates of breast cancer to nations such as Australia, Canada, and the United States, breast cancer risk climbs strongly, even within the lifetime of the migrant. Among older first-generation Japanese American women, for example, the incidence of breast cancer is almost seven times higher than that of older Japanese women living in Japan.

Environmental, dietary, and lifestyle factors are thought to play a role, but these have not been clearly identified. For example, dietary fat intake (especially animal fat) has been closely correlated with breast cancer death rates when comparisons are made among nations. But within the United States, women who ingest low-fat compared to high-fat diets do not appear to have lower breast cancer death rates, even when other risk factors are controlled. Experts disagree, however, on the influence of dietary fat on breast cancer, and the government is mounting the Women's Health Initiative, a $628 million trial involving 164,000 women. The study will help determine whether low-fat diets that are also high in fruits, vegetables, and grains lead to fewer cases of breast cancer.

Obesity, especially the "apple-shape" variety in which fat accumulates around the waist, increases the risk of breast cancer. Obesity is associated with higher blood insulin levels that promote the growth of breast cancer cells.

Animal studies have provided interesting results on the connection between exercise and breast cancer. Dr. Henry Thompson of the AMC Cancer Research Center in Denver, Colorado, has shown that 40 minutes of moderate-to-vigorous exercise, five days a week for 26 weeks, greatly reduces chemically-induced breast cancer in rats. Several other studies with animals have also led to the conclusion that exercise protects animals against chemically induced breast cancer.

Only a handful of human studies have been conducted, and findings are somewhat mixed. Of 12 major studies, 5 failed to establish a protective effect of physical activity against breast cancer. However, 7 other studies, especially those with good research designs, have supported this relationship.

For example, a review of the death records for some 25,000 women in Washington State revealed that those who had worked in physically demanding jobs had a low breast cancer risk. Another study of 6,888 women with breast cancer and 9,539 controls showed that women who had exercised vigorously on a near-daily basis between the ages of 14 and 22 years had a 50 percent reduction in breast cancer risk.

Dr. Rose Frisch of the Center for Population Studies in Cambridge, Massachusetts, studied the lifetime occurrence rate of breast cancer in 2,622 former female college athletes and 2,776 nonathletes. The nonathletes had an 86 percent higher risk for breast cancer than the former athletes throughout their lifetimes. Of interest is that the athletes were leaner and had a later age of menarche and an earlier age of menopause than the nonathletes.

Dr. Leslie Bernstein of the University of Southern California studied 545 premenopausal women with breast cancer and 545 controls. As shown in figure 4.2, the risk for breast cancer was reduced by more than half in women exercising more than 3.7 hours per week starting early in life.

A study of nearly 26,000 women in Norway showed that women who exercised at least four hours a week had 37 percent fewer breast cancers than women who spent their leisure hours reading, watching television, or engaging in other sedentary activities. Women whose jobs involved manual labor had 52 percent fewer breast cancers than women whose jobs kept them inactive. The researchers, led by Dr. Inger Thune of the University of Tromsö, also showed that the risk of breast cancer was lowest in lean women who exercised regularly (72 percent reduction in breast cancer risk).

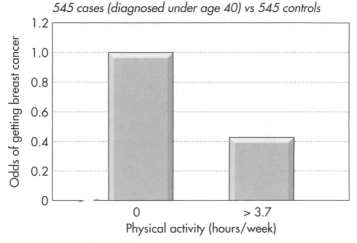

**Physical Activity and Reduced Risk of Breast Cancer**
*545 cases (diagnosed under age 40) vs 545 controls*

FIGURE 4.2    About four hours of exercise a week is associated with a reduced risk of breast cancer.

Although studies are mixed, there is good reason to continue examining the hypothesis that physical activity lowers breast cancer risk. As discussed earlier, the cumulative exposure to ovarian hormones is an important factor causing breast cancer. Women who exercise vigorously from childhood tend to have a later onset of menarche, may experience some missed menstrual cycles, and are generally leaner.

Leanness is important because increases in body fat elevate blood levels of certain types of estrogens. For this reason, Dr. Roy Shephard of the University of Toronto in Canada feels that reduction of body fat with regular exercise may be one of the chief protective mechanisms against breast cancer. Thus active athletic women may be protected from breast cancer because of the indirect effects of exercise on reducing exposure to their own female hormones.

## Other Female Reproductive Cancers

The critical role that the female hormone estrogen plays in cancer risk has also been shown for cancer of the uterus. Estrogen stimulates cell division within the lining of the uterus, increasing the risk for cancer cell development. As with breast cancer, uterine cancer risk is increased in women who are obese, who experience a late menopause, or who undergo prolonged estrogen therapy. Ovarian cancer risk is elevated in women who have never had children or have a family history of ovarian cancer.

Although more research is needed, there is evidence from five of six human studies that sedentary women are at substantially greater risk for female reproductive cancers than are those who are moderately to highly physically active. In one study, participation in college athletics was related to a reduced lifetime risk of both uterine and ovarian cancer. Nonathletes had more than 2.5 times the risk of female reproductive cancers than did former college athletes. Studies in Europe, China, and the United States have each shown that physical inactivity increases the risk for uterine cancer. Researchers from the National Cancer Institute have shown that physically inactive women may be at increased risk of endometrial cancer by virtue of their tendency to be obese.

## Prostate Cancer

The prostate is a walnut-sized gland tucked away under the bladder and adjacent to the rectum. It provides about a third of the fluid that propels sperm during sex. Nearly one-quarter million new cases of prostate cancer are experienced by American men each year, with rates about one-third higher for black men than for white men. About 40,000 men die each year from prostate cancer, which among cancers ranks second to lung cancer as a cause of death.

Early detection is critical in treating prostate cancer, and the American Cancer Society recommends that all men more than 40 years of age have a digital rectal examination each year, and for men more than 50, an annual prostate-specific antigen (PSA) blood test. Blood levels of PSA, an enzyme secreted only by the prostate, are related to the size of the prostate and can be an early detector of prostate cancer when combined with other tests.

More than 80 percent of all prostate cancers occur in men over age 65. Studies show that prostate cancer risk is 11 times higher among those who have a brother and a father with prostate cancer. The disease is more common in North America and northwestern Europe and is relatively rare in the Near East, Africa, Central America, and South America. For reasons not fully understood, African Americans have the highest rates for prostate cancer in the world. Prostate cancer rates in China and Japan, for example, are one-tenth those of U.S. blacks.

Migrant studies, as with colon and breast cancer, suggest that environmental and lifestyle factors play a role in prostate cancer. Chinese Americans and Japanese Americans have prostate cancer rates that are higher than those of their counterparts in Asia. Dr. Alice Whittemore of Stanford University has shown that high intake of dietary fat, especially animal fat, predicts increased risk of prostate cancer when different ethnic groups are compared.

There have been about 15 studies of physical activity and prostate cancer risk, and only about half of them have found inactivity to be a significant risk factor. There are even a few studies indicating that higher levels of physical activity predict increased risk of prostate cancer.

Researchers in Norway followed 53,242 men for an average of 16 years and found that risk of prostate cancer was reduced by more than half in those who walked during their work hours and also engaged in regular leisure-time exercise. This protective effect, however, was found only among men older than 60 years of age. These results are similar to those of a well-designed study of 17,719 college alumni by Dr. I-Min Lee of Harvard University. Risk of prostate cancer was reduced 47 percent in highly active versus sedentary men aged 70 years and older.

Dr. Susan Oliveria studied 12,975 men at the Cooper Clinic in Dallas, Texas, during 1970-1989. The men were given maximal exercise treadmill tests, divided into various fitness groups, and then tracked for development of prostate cancer over time. As shown in figure 4.3, men

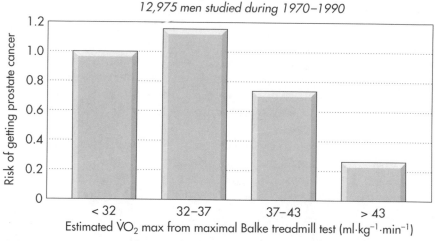

**Cardiorespiratory Fitness and Prostate Cancer**
*12,975 men studied during 1970–1990*

Risk of getting prostate cancer

Estimated $\dot{V}O_2$ max from maximal Balke treadmill test ($ml \cdot kg^{-1} \cdot min^{-1}$)

FIGURE 4.3    Increased aerobic fitness is associated with a lowered incidence of prostate cancer.

in the highest versus the lowest fitness group had a 74 percent reduced risk of developing prostate cancer. The men were also divided into different physical activity groups, and those exercising more than 1,000 calories per week had less than half the risk of prostate cancer of their more sedentary counterparts.

As with breast cancer, despite the inconsistent results from the few studies available, there is an attractive explanation for why regular physical activity may lower prostate cancer risk. Research suggests that higher levels of the male hormone testosterone may contribute to the development of prostate cancer. Animal studies have shown that prostate cancer can be provoked by injecting the animal with testosterone. As explained earlier, African Americans have the highest prostate cancer incidence rates in the world, which are almost entirely attributed to their higher testosterone levels (15 percent higher than for other American males). Antitestosterone therapy is the treatment of choice for advanced prostate cancer.

Most studies have demonstrated that testosterone concentrations are depressed in trained athletes. In other words, repeated bouts of exercise may lower blood levels of testosterone. The net effect is that highly active men may expose their prostate to less testosterone, reducing their risk of prostate cancer.

## EXERCISE AND TREATMENT OF CANCER

In the spring of 1988, Mark Conover surprised the U.S. marathoning community by winning the Olympic Marathon Trials in 2:12, a personal record by six minutes. Five years later, in the fall of 1993, Conover learned he had Hodgkin's disease, a type of lymphoma or cancer of the lymph nodes and other lymphoid tissues and cells. Risk factors for Hodgkin's disease are largely unknown, but in part involve reduced immune function and exposure to certain infectious agents. Chemotherapy and radiation are useful for most patients, and the overall five-year survival rate is 79 percent.

Drawing on the example of Fred Lebow, Conover decided to take an active and strong approach during his six months of therapy. Despite the nausea, fatigue, and hair loss caused by the treatments, Conover continued running 50 miles a week. "During this time, running proved to be my best friend, because it's a therapeutic, positive stress reliever," observed Conover.

After six months of therapy, Conover was told by medical personnel that his cancer was in remission. Two weeks before this discovery, Conover had run the Bay to Breakers race in San Francisco at a sub-5:20

minute per mile pace. Claimed Conover, "In a way, my cancer is a blessing. The things I'm feeling and thinking will deepen my soul. . . . And I can't lose. I'm already winning my most important fight."

---

### Can exercise help treat cancer once it is formed?

Probably not, but exercise by cancer patients is recommended to improve fitness, life quality, and morale.

---

In one of the few studies available, researchers followed 451 breast cancer patients for an average of five to six years while the patients reported their weekly levels of light, moderate, and vigorous physical activity. No link between exercise habits and survival from breast cancer could be measured. Animal research has determined that breast cancer risk is decreased by exercise during the earliest stages of cancer formation, but not after the cancer has become established.

Despite the limited research data, many experts still feel that moderate exercise may have several important benefits. According to Dr. Roy Shephard of the University of Toronto, "Exercise has an immediate mood-elevating effect, and thus can be of particular help to the cancer victim. It also stimulates appetite, and encourages the retention of muscle tissue. These effects should slow the clinical course of the disease, setting back the age at death, while also increasing the quality of the remaining years of life."

The Santa Barbara Athletic Club provides an exercise training program for cancer patients that are referred from a local cancer treatment center. The program has three components—aerobic, strength, and stretching/relaxation. Results from the program have shown that cancer patients can experience strong gains in upper- and lower-body strength and in aerobic fitness. Patients also reported improvement in their ability to engage in household tasks and recreational activities.

In Sweden, 200 cancer patients were assigned by researchers either to the "Starting Again" program or to the control condition. The program emphasized physical training, information, and coping skills. According to the researchers from the Karolinska Hospital in Stockholm, the patients in the program experienced greater "physical strength and a fighting spirit."

There is some concern that intensive exercise engaged in for extended periods of time may be detrimental. Both Drs. Leonard Cohen of the American Health Foundation and Laurie Hoffman-Goetz have advised that in animals, intense, forced, high-volume exercise enhances the spread of certain types of cancer. On the other hand, moderate exercise training acts to hold back the development of cancer, but has not been studied for its effect on treating cancer. A study by the American Cancer Society showed that heavy exercisers had higher death rates for various cancers than moderate exercisers.

Until more is known, it would be prudent to urge that all cancer patients exercise moderately each day while avoiding intensive exercise. Clinicians have been disturbed by the report of Fred Lebow's running a marathon as a cancer patient and by the example this has set for others like Mark Conover.

## REFERENCES

American Cancer Society. (1997). *Cancer facts & figures—1997*. Atlanta: American Cancer Society.

Ames, B.N., Shigenaga, M.K., & Hagen, T.M. (1993). Oxidants, antioxidants, and the degenerative diseases of aging. *Proceedings of the National Academy of Sciences, USA, 90*, 7915-7922.

Bernstein, L., Henderson, B.E., Hanisch, R., Sullivan-Halley, J., & Ross, R.K. (1994). Physical exercise and reduced risk of breast cancer in young women. *Journal of the National Cancer Institute, 86*, 1403-1408.

Durak, E.P., & Lilly, P.C. (1997, February). Cancer rehab in the health club. *Fitness Management*, 30-32.

Giovannucci, E., Ascherio, A., Rimm, E.B., Colditz, G.A., Stampfer, M.J., & Willett, W.C. (1995). Physical activity, obesity, and risk for colon cancer and adenoma in men. *Annals of Internal Medicine, 122*, 327-334.

Hackney, A.C. (1996). The male reproductive system and endurance exercise. *Medicine and Science in Sports and Exercise, 28*, 180-189.

Kramer, M.M., & Wells, C.L. (1996). Does physical activity reduce risk of estrogen-dependent cancer in women? *Medicine and Science in Sports and Exercise, 28*, 322-334.

Lee, I-M. (1994). Physical activity, fitness and cancer. In C. Bouchard, R.J. Shephard, & T. Stephens (Eds.), *Physical activity, fitness, and health: International proceedings and consensus statement*. Champaign, IL: Human Kinetics.

Lee, I-M. (1995). Exercise and physical health: Cancer and immune function. *Research Quarterly for Exercise and Sport, 66*, 286-291.

Nieman, D.C. (1995). *Fitness and sports medicine: A health-related approach*. Palo Alto, CA: Bull.

Oliveria, S.A., Kohl, H.W., Trichopoulos, D., & Blair, S.N. (1996). The association between cardiorespiratory fitness and prostate cancer. *Medicine and Science in Sports and Exercise, 28*, 97-104.

Shephard, R.J. (1995). Exercise and cancer: Linkages with obesity? *International Journal of Obesity*, *19* (Suppl. 4), S62-S68.

Thune, I., Brenn, T., Lund, E., and Gaard, M. (1997). Physical activity and the risk of breast cancer. *New England Journal of Medicine*, *336*, 1269-1275.

# Chapter 5

# STROKE

Moderate physical activity, such as frequent walking
and recreational activity, significantly reduces the risk of stroke,
and should be encouraged without restrictions.

**Dr. Goya Wannamethee, researcher, Royal Free Hospital School
of Medicine, London**

Although Americans could see for themselves that President Franklin
D. Roosevelt was failing rapidly, his personal physicians believed it was
necessary to keep from the public the truth about his health. World War
II was not yet won, and the President's aides would neither confirm nor
deny that he was ill and told no one, not even his family, that he had
serious heart problems and blood pressure as high as 260/150 mmHg.
Still, it came as a shock when President Roosevelt died of a massive
cerebral hemorrhage in 1945 at the age of 63. Most experts feel, however,
that his extremely high blood pressure was the major cause of his stroke.
On the other hand, it could be debated that the stress of being President
of the United States from 1933 to 1945 caused the increase in blood
pressure that led to Roosevelt's stroke.

## Pathology

The brain requires 20 to 25 percent of the heart's output of fresh blood
and 75 percent of the blood's glucose content. Two major artery systems
extend through the neck to disburse blood throughout the brain. Unlike
other organs, the brain cannot store energy, and if deprived of blood for
more than a few minutes, brain cells die from energy loss and certain
chemical interactions that are set in motion. The functions these brain
cells control—speech, vision, muscle movement, comprehension—die
with them.

Stroke is the common name for several disorders that occur within seconds or minutes after the blood supply to the brain is disturbed. The medical term is cerebrovascular disease or accident (CVA). The warning signals or symptoms of a stroke are sudden weakness or numbness of the face or limbs on one side of the body; loss of speech or comprehension; dimness or loss of vision, particularly in one eye; sudden, severe headaches with no known cause; and unexplained dizziness, unsteadiness, or sudden falls.

About 10 percent of strokes are preceded by "little strokes" called transient ischemic attacks or TIAs. Transient ischemic attacks can occur days, weeks, or even months before a major stroke. About 36 percent of people who have experienced TIAs will later have a stroke. Transient ischemic attacks occur when a blood clot temporarily clogs an artery, with the symptoms occurring rapidly and lasting only a short time (most less than five minutes).

Most strokes occur because the arteries in the brain become narrow from a buildup of plaque material or atherosclerosis. In fact, atherosclerosis is the underlying factor for both heart attacks and strokes (sometimes called "brain attacks"). Clots that form in the area of the narrowed brain blood vessels (called a thrombus) or ones that float in from other areas (an embolus) can then totally block the blood flow, causing the stroke. Three-fourths of strokes are caused by these clots that plug narrowed brain arteries.

Other strokes occur when a blood vessel in the brain or on its surface ruptures and bleeds (hemorrhagic stroke). Often the hemorrhage occurs when a spot in a brain artery has been weakened from atherosclerosis or high blood pressure. Hemorrhagic strokes are less common than those caused by clots, but are far more lethal.

## Prevalence

About 500,000 Americans experience a new or recurrent stroke each year. About 3 in 10 people who have a stroke die within a year, 6 in 10 within eight years. Each year, stroke kills about 150,000 people, accounting for 1 of every 15 U.S. deaths. It's the third largest cause of death, ranking behind diseases of the heart and cancer. Of those people who survive, one-half have long-term disabilities, needing help in caring for themselves or when walking.

The good news about stroke is that death rates have fallen dramatically during the better part of this century. Between 1950 and 1993 alone, stroke death rates fell an amazing 70 percent. Most of this decline is probably related to changes in lifestyle, according to Dr. Leslie Bronner of the Harvard School of Public Health. Migration studies, for example, show that when men born in Japan (who have very high stroke death rates) move to California, stroke death rates fall by more than half. This suggests, claims Bronner, "that environmental factors strongly influence the risk of stroke." Also, paralleling the decrease in stroke death rates have been reductions in the prevalence of three important stroke risk factors: high blood pressure, smoking, and high blood cholesterol levels.

## Prevention

The American Heart Association urges that the best way to prevent a stroke from occurring is to reduce the risk factors for stroke. "When stroke occurs, there can be severe losses in mental and bodily functions—if not death. That's why preventing stroke is so important," emphasizes the American Heart Association. And Dr. Bronner adds that "the outcome of a patient with a treated stroke may never be as good as that of someone in whom a stroke is prevented." This is because at present, no effective treatment for most forms of stroke has been established.

Seventy percent of all strokes occur in people with high blood pressure, making it the most important risk factor for stroke. In fact, stroke risk varies directly with blood pressure (see figure 5.1). What makes high blood pressure so important as a risk factor for stroke is that one in four Americans has it. And studies show that when high blood pressure is reduced, incidence of stroke falls with it.

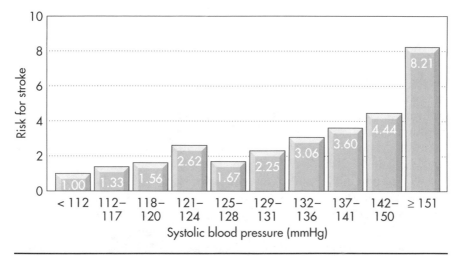

FIGURE 5.1   Systolic blood pressure and risk of stroke in 348,000 men over 12.5 years.

Additional risk factors that can be treated include cigarette smoking, obesity, excessive alcohol intake, high blood cholesterol levels, and physical inactivity. Several other stroke risk factors are categorized by the American Heart Association as unchangeable, including increasing age, being male, race, diabetes mellitus, prior stroke, and heredity. Strokes are more common in the southeastern United States, the so-called Stroke Belt, than in other areas of the United States.

Cigarette smoking is a major cause of stroke because it directly injures the blood vessel lining cells, increases the likelihood of clot formation, and acutely increases blood pressure. The risk of stroke for former smokers drops to the level of nonsmokers two to five years after quitting.

Incidence of stroke is strongly related to age, with the highest death rates found among people 85 years of age and over. The incidence of stroke is about 19 percent higher for men than for women, while African Americans have more than a 60 percent greater risk of death and disability from stroke than whites. The highest U.S. stroke death rates are found among African American males.

---

### If I exercise, am I less likely to have a stroke than if I don't exercise?

The American Heart Association does not feel there is sufficient evidence to rank physical inactivity as a primary risk factor for stroke.

---

The American Heart Association has categorized physical inactivity as a "secondary risk factor" because it affects the risk of stroke "indirectly by increasing the risk of heart disease (which is a primary risk factor for stroke)." In other words, the American Heart Association maintains that physical inactivity increases the risk for stroke indirectly through its influence on hypertension, obesity, and diabetes, but that insufficient data exist to support a direct effect of physical inactivity in and of itself.

Obesity is also ranked by the American Heart Association as a secondary risk factor because it increases the risk of stroke primarily through its adverse effects on other risk factors for cardiovascular disease (mainly high blood pressure, high blood cholesterol, and diabetes).

Table 5.1 shows that physical inactivity is related to several important stroke risk factors and that promotion of physical exercise is a good overall strategy for stroke prevention. As discussed in other chapters of this book, regular exercise tends to decrease body weight, lower blood pressure, increase high-density lipoprotein cholesterol levels, and improve diabetic control. There is increasing evidence that regular exercise also lowers the risk for blood clot formation. The end result is that physically active people should experience a lower risk for stroke.

TABLE 5.1

## Primary Prevention of Stroke, and Strategies for Reducing Risk

| Risk factor | Current prevalence | Strategies |
|---|---|---|
| High blood pressure (>140/90 mmHg) | 25% | Weight reduction, promotion of physical activity, reduced salt and alcohol intake |
| Smoking | 25% | Smoking cessation programs, physician counseling, nicotine patches, legislation |
| High serum cholesterol (>240 mg/dl) | 20% | Reduced saturated fat intake, weight reduction, physical activity (to raise HDL-C) |
| Obesity (>20% desirable weight) | 33% | Low-fat, low-energy diet, promotion of long-term physical activity, behavior change |
| Physical inactivity and irregular exercise habits | 60% | Work site fitness programs, community fitness facilities, physician counseling |
| Diabetes and impaired glucose tolerance | 11% | Weight reduction, promotion of physical activity, dietary improvement |

*If physical activity isn't a primary risk factor for stroke, why do you say exercise can help prevent strokes?*

A growing number of research studies have established a link between physical activity and decrease in stroke.

It is true that research on the relationship between physical inactivity and stroke is limited when compared to that for coronary heart disease. But according to Dr. Bronner, "The results from available studies are quite consistent." More than 15 major studies have now been published, and the more recent ones using the best research designs have reported a strong protective effect of regular exercise for both men and women.

Although some earlier studies in Finland, Sweden, and Italy did not report a protective effect, it is of interest that no study has found that regular exercise *increases* the risk for stroke.

It makes sense that if regular physical activity lowers coronary heart disease risk (a relationship that is very well established), stroke risk should also be lowered given the common underlying cause (athero-sclerosis). As shown in table 5.1, physical activity and fitness have a positive influence on blood pressure, diabetic control, and obesity, as well as other factors, including blood clot formation and perhaps even smoking habits (see chapter 12). With the lowering of risk factors, formation of atherosclerosis is less likely, translating to a reduced potential for clots and blocked brain arteries, or for the development of weak spots leading to hemorrhage.

The first research study providing evidence that physical activity may be related to a decreased risk of stroke was published in 1967 by Dr. Ralph Paffenbarger of Stanford University. Among 50,000 college alumni from the University of Pennsylvania and Harvard University, those men who were not varsity athletes during their college years had nearly a twofold increased risk of death from stroke compared to the varsity athletes.

In an extended follow-up of 17,000 alumni of Harvard University, Dr. Paffenbarger rated the men according to their leisure-time physical activity. Men in the lowest category of physical activity (those expend-ing less than 500 calories per week) died from stroke at a rate that was 1.7 times higher than for those who were most active (more than 2,000 calories per week). Another study of Dutch stroke patients and controls also established that men and women exercising the most during their leisure time exhibited the lowest risk of stroke (73 percent) when compared to those who were sedentary. However, even those reporting regular light activity during their leisure time (walking or cycling each week) experienced a 51 percent decreased risk of stroke.

Five studies published in the 1990s have provided the best evidence that physically active men and women experience fewer strokes. Dr. Roger Shinton of the University of Birmingham in Great Britain studied 105 stroke patients and 161 controls, and established that an increasing protection from stroke was experienced as the duration of exercise in earlier years increased. Risk of stroke fell 56 percent in those who had engaged in regular and vigorous exercise from ages 15 to 25, with some additional protection afforded those who exercised throughout adult-hood. As urged by Dr. Shinton, "This study adds weight to the evidence that exercise protects against the risk of stroke. Vigorous exercise in early adult life seems particularly beneficial, and lifelong continuation of exercise offers maximum protection."

Dr. Roger Abbott of the University of Virginia School of Medicine followed 7,530 men of Japanese ancestry living on the island of Oahu, Hawaii, for 22 years. Physical inactivity was found to be a strong risk factor for stroke caused by clots among nonsmoking middle-aged men (relative risk of 2.8) and for hemorrhagic stroke in older men ages 55-68 years (relative risk of 3.7) (see figure 5.2). According to Dr. Abbott, "For older middle-aged men, these data from Honolulu suggest that maintaining a physically active lifestyle may be one means of lowering the risk of stroke. In addition, it seems reasonable to expect that positive health behaviors and physical activity encouraged in younger men could improve their capacity to continue such behavior into their older years, where the benefits of reducing the risk of stroke are most pronounced."

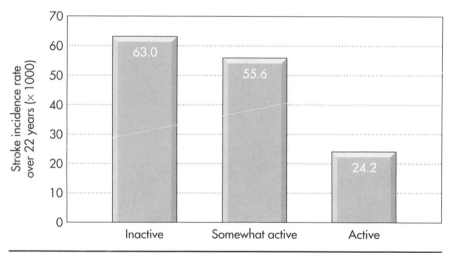

**FIGURE 5.2**   Stroke incidence rates for 7,530 Japanese men in Honolulu by physical activity habit.

---

### If I exercise more intensely, does the risk of stroke go down more?

Although more research is needed, there is evidence from several studies that while moderate physical activity is sufficient to lower the risk for stroke, further benefit is gained with increasing amounts and intensity of exercise.

---

The studies already reviewed in this chapter from Dr. Ralph Paffenbarger and Dr. Roger Abbott suggest that the more physical activity, the better, as far as stroke risk is concerned. Dr. Goya

Wannamethee of the Royal Free Hospital School of Medicine in London has provided the best evidence that a tight relationship between physical activity and stroke risk may exist. In other words, with increasing amounts of exercise, the stroke risk can be expected to drop in a steplike fashion.

Dr. Wannamethee followed 7,735 British middle-aged men for 9.5 years. A physical activity index was developed that rated the men according to the duration, frequency, and intensity of their activity habits. Men in the "vigorously active" category expended the most exercise calories, especially in sporting activities. As shown in figure 5.3, men who were moderately active experienced a 40 percent decrease in stroke risk, while those who were vigorously active had an even greater decrease (70 percent).

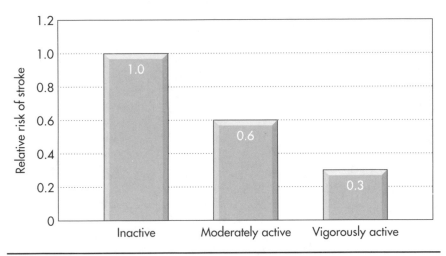

FIGURE 5.3   Risk of stroke for 7.735 British middle-aged men studied over 9.5 years by physical activity.

It should be stressed, however, that not all studies agree. Dr. Dan Kiely of the Boston University School of Medicine studied several thousand men and women from Framingham, Massachusetts, for 32 years and showed that older men exercising moderately experienced a 59 percent decrease in stroke risk. High levels of physical activity did not confer an additional benefit. No protective effect at all was found for women (i.e., whether they exercised or not had no effect on stroke risk). Dr. Kristian Lindsted of Loma Linda University in California followed 9,484 males for 26 years and found that moderately active men experienced a 22 percent decrease in stroke risk, with no significant protective effect measured for highly active men.

---

### Are the benefits of exercise in reducing stroke risk the same for women as for men?

Few studies have been conducted on women, and it is difficult at this time to say whether men and women respond differently when one considers physical activity and stroke risk.

---

Although the Framingham study reviewed in the previous paragraph showed that the women did not experience lower stroke risk with regular physical activity, a study by Dr. Ewa Lindenstrøm of Copenhagen provides an opposing viewpoint. Dr. Lindenstrøm followed 7,060 women aged 35 years and older for five years. She found that the risk of stroke in those exercising less than two hours a week intensely or four hours a week moderately was 45 percent higher than in those who were more active. Interestingly, the risk of stroke for the inactive women was just as strong as in those who smoked cigarettes.

## REFERENCES

Abbott, R.D., Rodriguez, B.L., Burchfiel, C.M., & Curb, J.D. (1994). Physical activity in older middle-aged men and reduced risk of stroke: The Honolulu Heart Program. *American Journal of Epidemiology, 139,* 881-893.

American Heart Association. (1995). *Heart and stroke facts.* Dallas: American Heart Association.

Bronner, L.L., Kanter, D.S., & Manson, J.E. (1995). Primary prevention of stroke. *New England Journal of Medicine, 333,* 1392-1400.

Kiely, D.K., Wolf, P.A., Cupples, L.A., Beiser, A.S., & Kannel, W.B. (1994). Physical activity and stroke risk: The Framingham Study. *American Journal of Epidemiology, 140,* 608-620.

Kohl, H.W., & McKenzie, J.D. (1994). Physical activity, fitness, and stroke. In C. Bouchard, R.J. Shephard, & T. Stephens (Eds.), *Physical activity, fitness, and health: International proceedings and consensus statement.* Champaign, IL: Human Kinetics.

Lindenstrøm, E., Boysen, G., & Nyboe, J. (1993). Lifestyle factors and risk of cerebrovascular disease in women: The Copenhagen City Heart Study. *Stroke, 24,* 1468-1472.

Shinton, R., & Sagar, G. (1993). Lifelong exercise and stroke. *British Journal of Medicine, 307,* 231-234.

Wannamethee, G., & Shaper, A.G. (1992). Physical activity and stroke in British middle aged men. *British Journal of Medicine, 304,* 597-601.

# Chapter 6

# DIABETES

Despite an important role of genetic factors,
non-insulin-dependent diabetes mellitus (NIDDM)
can be viewed as a largely preventable disease.

**Dr. JoAnn E. Manson, Harvard Medical School
and Brigham and Women's Hospital**

On July 30, 1921, Frederick Grant Banting, a research physician at the University of Toronto, and Charles Herbert Best, a medical student there, succeeded in isolating insulin from the pancreas of a dog. Within about one year, injections of insulin became available, and scientists began to think the disease could now be controlled. But it didn't turn out that way.

Researchers soon discovered that diabetes was not always caused by an absence of insulin in the body. In fact, some people with diabetes were found to have normal or even excessive amounts of insulin. And those diabetics who needed insulin injections still developed a host of disabling or lethal medical problems.

Diabetes gets it name from the ancient Greek work for siphon (a kind of tube) because early physicians noted that people with diabetes tended to be unusually thirsty and to urinate a lot. The "mellitus" part of the term is from the Latin version of the ancient Greek word for honey, used because doctors in centuries past diagnosed the disease by the sweet taste of the patient's urine.

## Pathogenesis

Diabetes impairs the body's ability to burn the fuel or glucose it gets from food for energy. Glucose is carried to the body's cells by the blood, but the cells need insulin, which is made by the pancreas (an organ just behind the stomach), to allow glucose to move inside. Without insulin, often likened to the key that unlocks the door, glucose accumulates in the blood, and then is dumped into the urine by the kidneys.

This sometimes happens because the cells of the pancreas that make insulin—the beta cells—are mostly or entirely destroyed by the body's own immune system (for reasons that are not fully understood). The patient then needs insulin injections to survive, and is diagnosed with insulin-dependent diabetes (IDDM). Another name for IDDM is type 1 diabetes. Because it usually starts in childhood or adolescence, IDDM used to be called juvenile-onset diabetes, but that term has been dropped because it is now known that this form of diabetes can begin at any age.

About 16 million Americans have diabetes, and 1,700 new cases are diagnosed every day. But only 5 to 10 percent of these are IDDM. The rest of the new cases are type 2 or noninsulin-dependent diabetes mellitus (NIDDM). In NIDDM, the person's beta cells do make insulin, but the patient's tissues aren't sensitive enough to the hormone, and use it inefficiently. In other words, there are plenty of keys to unlock the doors to allow glucose into the cells, but the locks (called insulin receptors) don't work very well or are few in number. This is called insulin resistance. As a result, both glucose and insulin can accumulate in the blood of patients with NIDDM.

Symptoms of IDDM typically appear abruptly and include excessive, frequent urination, insatiable hunger, and unquenchable thirst. Unexplained weight loss is also common, as are blurred vision, nausea and vomiting, weakness, drowsiness, irritability, and extreme fatigue.

Symptoms of NIDDM may include any or all those of IDDM, but are often overlooked because they tend to come on gradually and are less pronounced. Other symptoms may include tingling or numbness in the lower legs, feet, or hands; frequent and recurring skin, gum, or bladder infections; and cuts or bruises that are slow to heal. The onset of NIDDM is usually after age 30 and steadily increases with advancing age.

Measuring glucose levels in samples of the patient's blood is key to the diagnosis of both types of diabetes. The American Diabetes Association does not recommend that people have their serum glucose measured unless they are at high risk for diabetes or are experiencing symptoms. If the serum glucose is greater than or equal to 140 mg/dl on more than one occasion after an overnight, 12-hour fast, diabetes is diagnosed, especially when accompanied by the typical symptoms. A normal serum glucose is 70 to 115 mg/dl. Sometimes the physician will give the patient an oral glucose tolerance test (OGTT), especially when the blood glucose is between 115 and 140 mg/dl. This consists of a 75-gram glucose solution given after an overnight fast. If during the OGTT the one- and two-hour serum glucose levels are 200 mg/dl or higher, diabetes is diagnosed.

## Prognosis

People who have diabetes mellitus (the full medical term for diabetes) are vulnerable to many diseases due to the toxic effect of high blood glucose levels on blood vessels, nerves, and other tissues. Diabetes is the nation's leading cause of kidney failure and adult blindness and is a major cause of amputations of the toes, feet, and legs. About two-thirds of persons with diabetes have mild to severe forms of diabetic nerve damage, leading to impaired sensation in the feet or hands, delayed stomach emptying, and carpal tunnel syndrome. There is new evidence from the Mayo Clinic that diabetes increases the risk for Alzheimer's disease. More than three million hospitalizations each year are attributed to diabetes, exacting a heavy toll on this nation's health care system.

Since 1932, diabetes has ranked among the 10 leading causes of death in the United States. It is the cause of nearly 55,000 deaths annually and contributes to at least an additional 120,000 deaths. People with diabetes most often die of cardiovascular disease. Heart disease and stroke are two to four times more common among persons with diabetes, and are present in 75 percent of diabetes-related deaths. People with diabetes often have several risk factors for cardiovascular disease, including high blood pressure, elevated blood cholesterol and triglycerides, and low high-density lipoprotein cholesterol.

Recent studies have established that people with diabetes who need insulin must inject this hormone three or more times a day, measure blood glucose several times daily, and keep meticulous records and be very regular and consistent in their lifestyle in order to keep the blood glucose near normal levels and thus avoid the medical consequences.

## Prevention

According to the American Diabetes Association, IDDM and NIDDM have different causes, "yet two factors are important in both. First, you must inherit a predisposition to the disease. Second, something in your environment must trigger diabetes." Genes alone are not enough, because when one identical twin has IDDM, the other gets the disease at most only half the time. When one twin has NIDDM, the other's risk is at most three in four. However, NIDDM does run in families. For example, if one parent has NIDDM (diagnosed before age 50), the risk for the child's getting diabetes is one in seven. If both parents have NIDDM, the child's risk climbs to one in two.

## BOX 6.1
# The Diabetes Risk Test

Place a check in the box under "Yes" for each statement that is true for you. If the statement is not true for you, put a check in the box under "No." Total your score, adding up all the points for the boxes checked "Yes."

| | Yes | No |
|---|---|---|
| 1. I have been experiencing one or more of the following symptoms on a regular basis: | | |
| • excessive thirst | ☐ (3) | ☐ |
| • frequent urination | ☐ (3) | ☐ |
| • extreme fatigue | ☐ (1) | ☐ |
| • unexplained weight loss | ☐ (3) | ☐ |
| • blurry vision from time to time | ☐ (2) | ☐ |
| 2. I am over 30 years old. | ☐ (1) | ☐ |
| 3. My weight is equal to or above that listed in the chart below. | ☐ (2) | ☐ |
| 4. I am a woman who has had a baby weighing more than 9 pounds at birth. | ☐ (2) | ☐ |
| 5. I am of Native American, Hispanic, or African American descent. | ☐ (1) | ☐ |
| 6. I have a parent with diabetes. | ☐ (1) | ☐ |
| 7. I have a brother or sister with diabetes. | ☐ (2) | ☐ |

### Weight Chart (20% Over Maximum, Medium Frame)

| HEIGHT* | WEIGHT (lbs)* Women | Men | HEIGHT* | WEIGHT (lbs)* Women | Men |
|---|---|---|---|---|---|
| 4'9" | 127 | | 5'7" | 172 | 174 |
| 4'10" | 131 | | 5'8" | 176 | 179 |
| 4'11" | 134 | | 5'9" | 181 | 184 |
| 5'0" | 138 | | 5'10" | 186 | 190 |
| 5'1" | 142 | 146 | 5'11" | | 196 |
| 5'2" | 146 | 151 | 6'0" | | 202 |
| 5'3" | 151 | 155 | 6'1" | | 208 |
| 5'4" | 157 | 158 | 6'2" | | 214 |
| 5'5" | 162 | 163 | 6'3" | | 220 |
| 5'6" | 167 | 168 | | | |

*no shoes

### Scoring

**5 or more points:** You may be at high risk for or already have diabetes. See your doctor promptly to find out. If you experience symptoms later on, see your doctor immediately.
**3-4 points:** You probably are at low risk for diabetes (but still be concerned if you are over 30, overweight, or of African American, Hispanic, or Native American descent).

The American Diabetes Association feels that several environmental triggers for IDDM may include cold weather, certain types of viruses, or lack of breast-feeding. For NIDDM, family history is one of the strongest risk factors, along with increasing age, race (especially blacks, Mexican Americans, and Native Americans), obesity, other heart disease risk factors like high blood pressure and cholesterol, and gestational diabetes (women who get diabetes during the time they are pregnant). (See box 6.1 for the Diabetes Risk Test.)

Rates for NIDDM rise dramatically as the westernized lifestyle is adopted by people from developing societies. In the United States, approximately 85 percent of patients with NIDDM are obese at the time of diagnosis. The term "diabesity" has been used to describe this phenomenon. As shown in figure 6.1, the risk for developing NIDDM rises in direct relationship to the degree of obesity. In this 14-year study of 114,281 female nurses, after adjustment for age, body mass index (an obesity index calculated by dividing the body weight in kilograms by the height in meters squared) was the dominant predictor of risk for NIDDM. Women who gained weight during the study increased their risk for NIDDM, while those who lost weight decreased their risk. According to Dr. Graham Colditz, the lead investigator of the study from the Harvard School of Public Health, "These data strongly suggest that women can minimize the risk for diabetes by achieving a lean body build as a young adult and avoiding even modest weight gain throughout life."

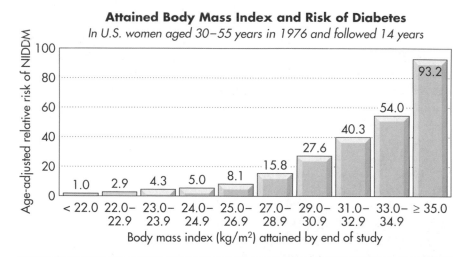

FIGURE 6.1   The relative risk of NIDDM rises strongly with the body mass index attained as an adult.

# LIFESTYLE TREATMENT OF DIABETES

Treatment for either type of diabetes seeks to accomplish what the human body normally does naturally: maintain a proper balance between glucose and insulin. Food makes the blood glucose level rise while insulin and exercise make it fall. The trick is to juggle the three factors to keep the blood glucose within a narrow range.

Since there is no cure for IDDM, treatment is lifelong. For the IDDM, in order keep the blood glucose within narrow limits and avoid the medical complications, a regular and consistent lifestyle must be followed. Eating times, amounts and types of foods, and physical activity should be consistent from one day to the next. Blood glucose should be measured several times a day, and multiple insulin injections or treatment with an insulin pump is necessary.

Results from a major multicenter study (the Diabetes Control and Complications Trial Research Group) have shown that when IDDM patients keep their blood glucose levels under tight control through intensive care, fewer medical complications develop. As Dr. Edward S. Horton, of the University of Vermont, and a former president of the American Diabetes Association, has emphasized, "Diabetes can be a deadly disease. But with the help of modern medicine and their own efforts, many patients can lead long, active, and relatively healthy lives."

Most experts recommend that a staged approach to diabetic treatment be followed for NIDDM patients. Because the vast majority are obese, weight loss through a healthy diet (i.e., low in fat, with an emphasis on carbohydrates and fiber) and exercise is first recommended. If diet, exercise, and weight loss fail to lower blood glucose levels (most often due to patient noncompliance with the recommended lifestyle changes), the physician may decide to add an oral sulfonylurea drug, insulin, or both. Sulfonylurea drugs are used only for NIDDM, mainly for patients whose diabetes is judged to be less severe. Insulin is the usual choice for advanced NIDDM cases.

Experts have estimated that with optimum long-term diet and exercise therapy, and achievement of ideal body weight, only about 1 in 10 NIDDM patients would require any kind of medication. In other words, 90 percent of NIDDM is thought to be preventable and treatable through improved lifestyle habits.

The single most important objective for the obese person with NIDDM is to achieve and maintain a desirable body weight. Weight reduction reduces serum glucose and improves insulin sensitivity while also favorably influencing several heart disease risk factors. Persons with diabetes who are at high risk for death from heart disease and face a future laden with medical complications from high blood glucose levels have much to gain from losing weight.

Figure 6.2 summarizes how quickly weight loss through a healthy diet and exercise program can influence NIDDM and heart disease risk factors. In this study, 652 NIDDM patients attended the Pritikin Longevity Center 26-day residential program. The group included 212 patients taking insulin and 197 taking oral hypoglycemic agents. The remaining 243 were taking no diabetic medication but had a fasting glucose level above 140 mg/dl. During the 26-day program, the NIDDM patients were involved in daily aerobic exercise, primarily walking (building up to two one-hour walks each day). Patients were also placed on a high-carbohydrate, high-fiber, low-fat, low-cholesterol, and low-salt diet. Of dietary calories, less than 10 percent were obtained from fat. The diet contained 35 to 40 grams of dietary fiber per 1,000 calories—a very high amount according to most standards. The average patient lost about 10 pounds during the program and experienced strong reductions in blood pressure, fasting glucose, total cholesterol, and triglycerides. Of patients on insulin, 39 percent were able to stop therapy, and 71 percent of patients on oral agents also had their medication discontinued.

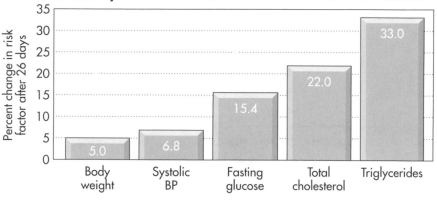

**Effects of Healthy Diet and Exercise on CHD Risk Factors in Diabetics**

FIGURE 6.2   Diet and aerobic exercise are effective in controlling NIDDM and reducing risk factors.

Because of the way this study was designed, it is not possible to sort out which lifestyle factor—exercise, weight loss, or improved diet—was most responsible for the impressive results. Although the Pritikin diet has been criticized as being unusually restrictive (and hard to continue once the program stops), Dr. James Barnard, lead investigator of the study from UCLA, feels that "even though the optimal diet has not been determined, the results of this study indicate a real need for strong emphasis on lifestyle modification consisting of both diet and exercise in the treatment of NIDDM."

There has been considerable debate over the past half century regarding the diet best suited for persons with diabetes. Table 6.1 shows that there has been a progression of change toward less and less dietary fat and more and more carbohydrate, with an emphasis today that the diet should be individualized for each patient. The primary goals of the diabetic diet for NIDDM patients are to lower blood glucose and lipids, blood pressure, and body weight (when necessary). For these reasons, NIDDM patients should follow a healthy and varied diet, with an emphasis on controlling saturated fats.

## TABLE 6.1
## Changes in the Diabetic Diet (Percentage of Total Calories)

| Year | % Carbohydrate | % Protein | % Fat |
| --- | --- | --- | --- |
| Before 1921 | Low calorie | Low calorie | Low calorie |
| 1921 | 20 | 10 | 70 |
| 1950 | 40 | 20 | 40 |
| 1971 | 45 | 20 | 35 |
| 1986 | Up to 60 | 12-20 | <30 |
| 1994 | Individualized | 10-20 | Individualized <10% saturated fats |

---

### If I exercise, will my chances of developing diabetes be lowered?

Although more study is needed, the best studies have provided compelling evidence that active individuals are at 30-50 percent lower risk for NIDDM than are their inactive peers.

---

Researchers have established that NIDDM is less common in physically active compared to inactive societies. Also, as populations have become more sedentary, the incidence of NIDDM has been observed to increase; NIDDM, for example, is unusually common among some South Pacific and native American tribes who have adopted the sedentary habits of the Western world. However, experts point out that other environmental and lifestyle factors are probably involved, including changes in body weight and dietary habits.

More impressive are data from five recent major studies that have followed large groups of men and women for extended periods of time to measure the influence of physical activity and inactivity on the risk of developing NIDDM. Each of the five studies has provided convincing support for the role of regular physical activity in the prevention of NIDDM.

The first study was published in the summer of 1991 by a group of researchers led by Dr. Ralph Paffenbarger from the Stanford University School of Medicine. Nearly 6,000 male alumni of the University of Pennsylvania were followed for about 14 years. Leisure-time physical activity was measured and expressed as calories expended per week for walking, stair climbing, and sport. Noninsulin-dependent diabetes developed in 202 men; and the important finding was that for each 500 calorie per week increase in activity expenditure, the risk of NIDDM was reduced by 6 percent. For men who were both obese and inactive, the likelihood of developing NIDDM was four times greater than for lean and active men. The protective effect of physical activity was especially strong for men at highest risk for NIDDM, as shown in figure 6.3. As emphasized by Dr. Horton in an accompanying editorial, "Regular physical activity is an important component of a healthy lifestyle for all of us, but it may be particularly important for those at increased risk for chronic diseases such as NIDDM, hypertension, and hyperlipidemia."

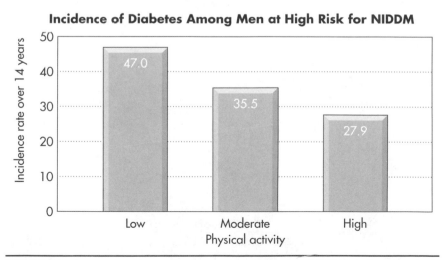

FIGURE 6.3    Leisure-time physical activity is protective against NIDDM, especially in high-risk men.

Other studies have provided firm support for the idea that regular exercise helps to lower the risk of developing NIDDM for both men and women. Dr. JoAnn Manson of the Harvard Medical School and Brigham and Women's Hospital in Boston followed 87,252 nurses for eight years. Women who exercised vigorously at least once a week experienced a 33 percent reduction in risk of NIDDM. These results are very similar to the findings of Dr. Manson's five-year study of 21,271 male physicians. Subjects who exercised regularly experienced a 36 percent reduction in risk of NIDDM, with the risk found to be lowest among those exercising most frequently. As with the Stanford study, the benefits of exercise "were most pronounced among the obese, who have the highest risk of NIDDM," observed Dr. Manson.

In Great Britain, 7,735 men were followed for nearly 13 years. The risk of developing NIDDM was found to be reduced by more than 50 percent among the most physically active men as compared to their relatively inactive peers. In Finland, men who exercised at a moderately intense level for more than 40 minutes per week reduced their risk of developing NIDDM by 64 percent compared to men who did not exercise. In Hawaii, a six-year study of 6,815 Japanese American men came to a similar conclusion. As depicted in figure 6.4, the rate of developing NIDDM was lowest among the most active men, even after adjustment for age, obesity, family history, and other factors known to influence the risk of diabetes.

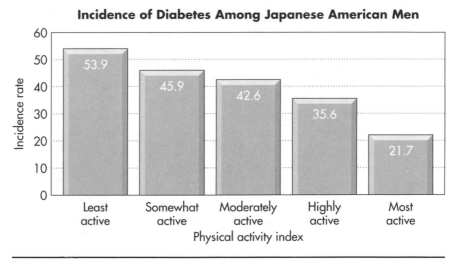

**Incidence of Diabetes Among Japanese American Men**

**FIGURE 6.4**   The incidence of diabetes (over 6 years) was highest among those exercising least.

*My doctor said that because of my weight and poor diet I'm at risk for developing diabetes. What role does physical activity play in this whole mix?*

While both are important risk factors for NIDDM, obesity is felt by most experts to rank above physical inactivity. More research is needed to determine whether a high-fat, low-fiber diet is a significant risk factor for the development of NIDDM.

There is overwhelming evidence that obesity is a major risk factor for NIDDM. In severely obese populations, such as the Pima Indians and Nauruans, the prevalence of NIDDM is the highest worldwide. Long-term studies of large groups of people have consistently shown that obesity is a strong predictor of the development of NIDDM in women and men.

Obesity, especially upper-body or abdominal obesity, is associated with insulin resistance, that is, a decreased ability of the body to respond to the action of insulin as well as a reduced number of insulin receptors. A growing number of studies have shown that the risk of NIDDM climbs in direct proportion to the increase in the waist-to-hip ratio (i.e., when the abdominal girth approaches or exceeds the hip girth). When the abdominal fat is lost, the insulin resistance is reduced, and blood glucose levels often return to normal.

According to Dr. Manson, the estimated reduction in the risk of NIDDM associated with maintaining desirable body weight compared with being obese is 50 to 75 percent—considerably higher than the 30 to 50 percent reduction in risk associated with regular moderate or vigorous exercise versus a sedentary lifestyle.

Few studies have been conducted on the role of diet in the development of NIDDM. Diet is regarded as an important component of treatment, but whether low-fat, high-fiber diets help prevent NIDDM is largely unknown. In one six-year study of more than 65,000 nurses, researchers from the Harvard School of Public Health showed that the risk of developing diabetes was 2.5 times greater in those using refined and processed grain products (low in dietary fiber) compared to those using grains in a minimally refined form (high in fiber).

The concept that physical activity is beneficial for people with diabetes is not new. It was promoted as a valuable adjunct to diabetic control in 600 A.D. by Chao Yuan-Fang, a prominent Chinese physician of the Sui dynasty. Even after the isolation of insulin in 1922, exercise was considered as one of the three cornerstones of therapy for IDDM patients, along with diet and insulin. Although the concept that physical activity is beneficial for individuals with diabetes is centuries old, there is still considerable controversy about it.

---

### How does exercise affect my insulin and blood glucose levels?

During exercise, to maintain a constant blood glucose level, the blood concentration of insulin drops to counter the "insulin-like" effect of muscle contraction. Thus the working muscle can take in glucose even though little insulin is present. Another hormone from the pancreas, glucagon, stimulates the liver to release glucose to provide fuel for the muscles.

---

The pancreas secretes two hormones, insulin and glucagon, to help maintain blood glucose levels. During rest, when blood glucose levels rise after a meal, insulin is secreted to help move the glucose into the body cells. Receptors on the body cells require that insulin be present before glucose can enter. On the other hand, when blood glucose levels drop, glucagon is secreted to increase blood glucose levels by stimulating the breakdown of liver glycogen (i.e., stored carbohydrate).

During exercise, blood insulin levels drop, while blood glucagon levels increase. These changes take place to counterbalance the insulin-like effect of muscle contraction. As the muscles contract during exercise, they do not require much insulin to transport glucose into the working cells. The exercising muscle may increase the uptake of glucose 7- to 20-fold during the first 30 to 40 minutes, depending on the intensity.

In addition, the insulin receptors become more "sensitive" to the lower amount of insulin present during exercise. This improvement in insulin receptor sensitivity can last for many hours after the exercise bout is over, even for as long as two days if the exercise was of long duration and high intensity.

---

### Of what value is regular exercise for the person with insulin-dependent diabetes?

Although regular exercise by the IDDM patient leads to reduced insulin requirements, overall glucose control is not improved. However, there are many other potential benefits from regular exercise, including improved control of cardiovascular disease risk factors, enhanced fitness, and elevated psychological well-being.

---

For nearly 50 years, researchers have known that regular exercise will reduce the insulin requirements of well-controlled IDDM patients by 30-50 percent. It appears, however, that each bout of exercise leads to an improvement in insulin sensitivity that lasts for only one or two days before falling back to pre-exercise levels. In other words, the muscles need regular exercise to maintain an enhanced insulin sensitivity. The net result is that a given amount of insulin following exercise is more effective in causing glucose uptake by the cells. The IDDM patient who exercises regularly will need smaller-than-normal insulin doses, or will have to increase food intake (see next section).

Although regular exercise leads to reduced insulin requirements for the person with IDDM, studies have failed to show that long-term glucose control is improved, according to the American Diabetes Association (ADA). The ADA still feels that IDDM patients have much to gain from exercising regularly "because of the potential to improve cardiovascular fitness and psychological well-being and for social interaction and recreation."

---

### Are there potential risks for the individual with insulin-dependent diabetes who initiates an exercise program?

Physical exercise is not without risks to individuals with IDDM. The principal risk is low blood glucose, but some IDDM patients with high initial blood glucose levels can raise them even more with exercise. There is also the potential that diabetic complications (e.g., heart disease, foot problems, retinal disease, etc.) can be worsened if the patient does not take the appropriate precautions.

---

The ADA has urged that "safe participation in all forms of exercise, consistent with an individual's lifestyle, should be a primary goal for people with IDDM." However, the ADA adds that "physical exercise is not without risks to IDDM individuals."

While nondiabetic individuals usually experience little change in blood glucose levels during exercise, patients with IDDM may see an increase (i.e., hyperglycemia) or a decrease (hypoglycemia) depending on their initial levels.

Patients with IDDM who have very high blood glucose levels (above 250 mg/dl) with ketones in their urine can experience a rapid rise in blood glucose upon starting exercise, as well as the development of ketosis. For this reason, people with IDDM should postpone exercise until they have gotten their blood glucose under control through proper diet and insulin therapy.

For most IDDM patients who begin exercising, the principal risk is hypoglycemia. The ADA cautions that "many variables, including fitness, duration and intensity of exercise, and time of exercise regarding insulin administration and meals will affect the metabolic response to exercise." Hypoglycemia is most likely to occur when the exercise is prolonged and/or intense, when the blood glucose prior to exercise was near normal, and when the exercise takes place shortly after insulin injection into a muscle used during the bout.

To avoid hypoglycemia during or after exercise, a regular pattern of exercise and diet should be adopted, with frequent blood glucose measurements to test the body's response. Each individual with IDDM is unique, and each will need to discover for him or herself the best schedule to follow to keep the blood glucose under tight control. Exercise should be performed at the same convenient time every day, at approximately the same intensity and for the same amount of time. Morning appears to be preferable to evening for most persons with IDDM because episodes of delayed hypoglycemia may occur during sleep following late-day exercise.

Exercise should not be performed at the time of peak insulin effect (i.e., within one hour after an injection of short-acting insulin). Because of the insulin-like effect of exercise, the person with IDDM initiating an exercise program will have to reduce insulin dosage (by about one-third) and/or increase food intake. Insulin injections should not be at sites of the body that will be exercised soon thereafter (e.g., thighs that will be used in running or cycling).

During prolonged physical activity, 60 to 120 calories of carbohydrate (i.e., the amount found in one to two cups of most sport drinks) is recommended for each 30 minutes. A meal one to three hours before exercise is recommended, and fluids should be taken during and after exercise to avoid dehydration. A carbohydrate snack is recommended soon after unusually strenuous exercise.

Several of the long-term complications of diabetes may be worsened by exercise. Vigorous exercise may precipitate heart attack when there is underlying coronary heart disease, a common medical problem in diabetics. Patients with IDDM who are over 40 years of age, individuals who have had diabetes for 10 years or more, or those with established complications should first undergo a thorough medical exam that includes a graded exercise stress test.

There is some concern that large and sustained increases in blood pressure during heavy exertion may accelerate the development of eye or kidney problems in persons with IDDM. Until more is known, IDDM patients with these complications are cautioned to avoid sustained heavy exercise such as vigorous weight lifting or prolonged, intense aerobic activity.

Patients with IDDM who have nerve and blood vessel damage in their feet and legs should be particularly careful to avoid cuts, blisters, and pounding exercises of the lower extremities (e.g., running, high-impact aerobic dance, etc.). Good footwear, careful foot hygiene, and regular inspection are necessary.

---

### Can I compete in sports if I have insulin-dependent diabetes?

With appropriate medical support and education, children, adolescents, and adults with IDDM can perform athletically. Careful attention must be given to blood glucose monitoring within the context of a carefully planned and regular schedule of medication, training, and eating.

---

According to Dr. David Robbins of the University of Vermont College of Medicine, "Not long ago, the terms 'diabetic' and 'athlete' seemed mutually exclusive." Today, partly because of the advent of blood glucose self-monitoring and the recognition that exercise brings multiple benefits, many diabetic athletes have entered the sporting arena with the approval and support of their physicians. Nationally known athletes with diabetes have included Ty Cobb, Jackie Robinson, Catfish Hunter, Bobby Clarke, Scott Verplank, and Wade Wilson. Adds Dr. Robbins, "So long as diabetic athletes understand the interactions among diet, exertion, and insulin and are aware of their unique reactions to exercise, they can safely engage in almost any sport or activity."

As mentioned in the previous section, strenuous exercise is not recommended for some people with IDDM, especially those with medical complications. For the majority of diabetic patients, however, participation in competitive sport, in collaboration with a physician, is feasible and beneficial. According to Dr. Piers Blackett of the University of Oklahoma Health Sciences Center, "Participation in sports during childhood may enhance self-image, provide a sense of accomplishment, and lead to social interactions that are conducive to optimal emotional development." Exercise can also serve as an incentive for children and adolescents to attain tighter control of their blood glucose.

No two individuals with diabetes respond to exercise in exactly the same way. With the guidance of a physician, the athlete with IDDM, through a process of trial and error, can discover what adjustments in carbohydrate, insulin dosage, or a combination of the two work best. This process requires frequent blood glucose monitoring and correction.

According to Dr. Robbins, "The most appropriate exercises for diabetic patients involve predictable levels of physical expenditure. Among the patients in our practice are competitive cyclists, marathon runners, cross-country skiers, and triathletes, all of whom maintain control by frequent self-testing and adjustment before, during, and after training sessions and events. These sports are compatible with good diabetic control because they involve predetermined distances, duration, and intensity of competition, as well as predictable frequency. Therefore, these activities permit the athlete to anticipate his or her physical needs."

---

## What does exercise do for people with noninsulin-dependent diabetes?

For most individuals with NIDDM, regular exercise improves glycemic control, reduces certain heart disease risk factors, improves psychological well-being, and promotes weight reduction.

---

The major aim of therapy for NIDDM patients is to improve insulin sensitivity through appropriate use of diet, exercise, and weight reduction. In contrast to results with IDDM patients, regular exercise by persons with NIDDM does lead to improved long-term diabetic control. For obese NIDDM patients on insulin, exercise and weight reduction can reduce insulin requirements by up to 100 percent. Improved glucose control has been shown for both middle-aged and elderly NIDDM patients who exercise regularly, due in part to the frequent lowering of the blood glucose level and enhancement of insulin sensitivity with each exercise session.

According to the ADA, "Patients who are most likely to respond favorably are those with mildly to moderately impaired glucose tolerance and hyperinsulinemia." The ADA cautions that the benefits of exercise typically outweigh the risks if attention is given to "minimizing potential exercise complications." All individuals with NIDDM who are about to start an exercise program should have a thorough medical exam to uncover previously undiagnosed complications due to diabetes.

In one seven-year study of 548 diabetes patients at the University of Pittsburgh, regular physical activity was shown to have a beneficial effect in extending longevity. Although there has been some concern that NIDDM patients are at high risk for heart attack during exercise because of their multiple risk factors, this study established that "activity is not detrimental with regard to mortality, and may in fact provide a beneficial effect in terms of longevity," according to Dr. Claudia Moy, who was the lead investigator.

---

### Is there a "best" exercise program for people with diabetes?
The exercise recommendations for people with diabetes are similar to those for healthy adults.

---

For most diabetic individuals who have been given medical clearance to begin exercising, near-daily physical activity, for 20 to 45 minutes, at a moderate to somewhat hard intensity level, is recommended. A high frequency of exercise is essential since the residual effects of an acute exercise bout on glucose tolerance last for only one or two days. Also, for an obese person with NIDDM, near-daily activity will help ensure that an adequate number of calories are expended to assist in weight loss.

Exercise sessions of less than 20 minutes' duration appear to have little benefit for diabetic control, while sessions lasting more than 45 minutes increase the risk of hypoglycemia. According to Dr. Barry Baun of the University of California at Berkeley, low-intensity exercise (50 percent of $\dot{V}O_2max$) is just as effective as high-intensity exercise (75 percent of $\dot{V}O_2max$) in enhancing insulin sensitivity in persons with diabetes as long as the caloric expenditure is equalized by increasing the duration of the low-intensity exercise bouts.

Since most people with diabetes are poorly conditioned, an easy start to the exercise program, with gradual progression, is advised. Aerobic, endurance-type activities involving large muscle groups, such as cycling, brisk walking, and swimming, are recommended. Weight-training exercises designed to improve muscle endurance through high repetitions with moderate weight will help avoid high blood pressure responses. Each exercise session should begin with an appropriate warm-up and cooldown period.

Unfortunately, studies have shown that the majority of people with diabetes do not exercise regularly, and they tend to exercise less than people who do not have diabetes. According to national data compiled by Dr. Earl Ford of the Centers for Disease Control, only about one in three people with diabetes reports exercising regularly, and less than one in five burns 2,000 calories or more per week in exercise. "The data suggest that, as is the case for the general population, ample room for improvement exists in the exercise habits of Americans with diabetes," Dr. Ford states in his summary.

Most experts feel that health care providers play a key role in encouraging their patients with diabetes to exercise. However, in one study, only 25 percent of people with diabetes reported receiving specific guidelines about exercise from any type of health care professional.

# REFERENCES

Barnard, R.J., Jung, T., & Inkeles, S.B. (1994). Diet and exercise in the treatment of NIDDM. *Diabetes Care, 17,* 1469-1472.

Burchfiel, C.M., Sharp, D.S., Curb, J.D., Rodriguez, B.L., Hwang, L-J., Marcus, E.B., & Yano, K. (1995). Physical activity and incidence of diabetes: The Honolulu Heart Program. *American Journal of Epidemiology, 141,* 360-368.

Colditz, G.A., Willett, W.C., Rotnitzky, A., & Manson, J.E. (1995). Weight gain as a risk factor for clinical diabetes mellitus in women. *Annals of Internal Medicine, 122,* 481-486.

Ford, E.S., & Herman, W.H. (1995). Leisure-time physical activity patterns in the U.S. diabetic population. *Diabetes Care, 18,* 27-33.

Gudat, U., Berger, M., & Lefèbvre, P.J. (1994). Physical activity, fitness, and non-insulin-dependent (type II) diabetes mellitus. In C. Bouchard, R.J. Shephard, & T. Stephens (Eds.), *Physical activity, fitness, and health: International proceedings and consensus statement* (pp. 669-683). Champaign, IL: Human Kinetics.

Helmrich, S.P., Ragland, D.R., Leung, R.W., & Paffenbarger, R.S. (1991). Physical activity and reduced occurrence of non-insulin-dependent diabetes mellitus. *New England Journal of Medicine, 325,* 147-152.

Leibson, C.L., Rocca, W.A., Hanson, V.A., Cha, R., Kokmen, E., O'Brien, P.C., & Palumbo, P.J. (1997). Risk of dementia among persons with diabetes mellitus: A population-based cohort study. *American Journal of Epidemiology, 145,* 301-308.

Lynch, J., Helmrich, S.P., Lakka, T.A., Kaplan, G.A., Cohen, R.D., Salonen, R., & Salonen, J.T. (1996). Moderately intense physical activities and high levels of cardiorespiratory fitness reduce the risk of non-insulin-dependent diabetes mellitus in middle-aged men. *Archives of Internal Medicine, 156,* 1307-1314.

Manson, J.E., Rimm, E.B., Stampfer, M.J., Colditz, G.A., Willett, W.C., Krolewski, A.S., Rosner, B., Hennekens, C.H., & Speizer, F.E. (1991). Physical activity and incidence of non-insulin-dependent diabetes mellitus in women. *Lancet, 338,* 774-778.

Manson, J.E., & Spelsberg, A. (1994). Primary prevention of non-insulin-dependent diabetes mellitus. *American Journal of Preventive Medicine, 10,* 172-184.

Perry, I.J., Wannamethee, A.G., Walker, M.K., Thomson, A.G., Whincup, P.H., & Shaper, A.G. (1995). Prospective study of risk factors for development of non-insulin dependent diabetes in middle aged British men. *British Medical Journal, 310,* 560-564.

Robbins, D.C., & Carleton, S. (1989). Managing the diabetic athlete. *The Physician and Sportsmedicine, 17* (12), 45-54.

Salmerón, J., Manson, J.E., Stampfer, M.J., Colditz, G.A., Wing, A.L., & Willett, W.C. (1997). Dietary fiber, glycemic load, and risk of non-insulin-dependent diabetes mellitus in women. *Journal of the American Medical Association, 277,* 472-477.

U.S. Preventive Services Task Force. (1996). *Guide to clinical preventive services* (2nd ed.). Alexandria, VA: International Medical Publishing, Inc.

Young, J.C. (1995). Exercise prescription for individuals with metabolic disorders. Practical considerations. *Sports Medicine, 19,* 43-53.

# Chapter 7

# OSTEOPOROSIS

Bone health is promoted through regular weight-bearing
physical activities that use muscular strength and power,
and exert force on the skeleton above normal amounts.

### President's Council on Physical Fitness and Sports

Jacqueline Wallace of Phoenix sat enjoying the December 1993 holiday
at her son's home. But when she stood up and took a step, her holiday
took a turn for the worse. Mrs. Wallace, aged 84 years, fell and fractured
her hip. "My foot dragged a little, not exactly a stumble," she recalls. "I
don't know whether the bone broke because I fell, or I fell because the
bone broke."

Mrs. Wallace's fracture was one of 1.5 million—including 336,000 hip
fractures—reported that year in the United States. The cause? Osteoporosis, a bone-weakening disease that develops gradually and
makes bones so fragile that they fracture under normal use. Osteoporosis, sometimes called "brittle bone disease," gets its name from the Latin
term for "porous bones." The sites most commonly affected are the
spine, hips, and forearms.

## Prevalence

Roughly 25 million Americans, primarily women, have this disease. The
cost of osteoporosis will exceed $60 billion by the year 2000. The World
Summit of Osteoporosis Societies estimates that as many as 200 million
people worldwide have osteoporosis. And if present trends continue,
the prevalence of osteoporosis is expected to double by the year 2020.

Osteoporosis is a "silent disease" that progresses without any out-
ward sign, sometimes for decades, until a fracture occurs. These broken
bones often result from a minor fall or bump that would not normally

cause a break. People may lose height from collapsed spinal vertebrae (called "dowager's hump") without realizing they have osteoporosis.

After women go through menopause, nearly one in three will develop osteoporosis (see figure 7.1). Among persons who live to age 90, 33 percent of women and 17 percent of men will experience hip fractures. An estimated 12 to 20 percent of elderly people who have hip fractures die of complications within a year of the fracture, while 50 percent of the survivors require some help with daily living activities. Obviously, osteoporosis is an important public health problem, exacting an enormous economic and medical burden on the elderly population.

**Cross-Sections of Normal and Osteoporotic Bone**

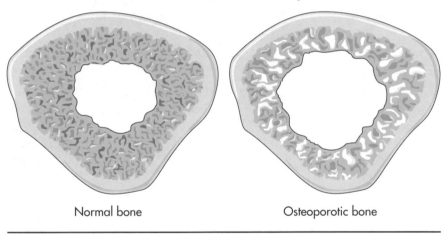

Normal bone                    Osteoporotic bone

FIGURE 7.1    Osteoporosis is characterized by a loss of normal bone mass.

## Pathogenesis

Bone is not a hard and lifeless structure. It is, in fact, a complex living tissue that provides structural support for muscles, protects vital organs, and stores the calcium essential for bone density and strength. The body's 206 dynamic, living bones renew themselves throughout life by means of a continual breakdown-buildup process known as remodeling. In remodeling, complex chemical signals prompt bone cells called osteoclasts to break down and remove old bone, and others called osteoblasts to deposit new bone.

During puberty, rapid increases in bone growth and density occur, with peak bone density achieved between the ages of 20 and 30. Once peak bone mass is reached, osteoclast and osteoblast activity remain in balance until about age 45 to 50, when osteoclast activity becomes greater and adults begin to slowly lose bone mass. At menopause, women normally have an accelerated loss of bone mineral mass for several years as they lose the protective effect of estrogen.

About 90 percent of the adult bone mineral content is deposited by the end of adolescence, and this process is affected by both genetic and lifestyle factors. Most experts feel that the period between age 9 and 20 years is critical in building up an optimal bone density as a safeguard against the inevitable losses that will occur with aging. The National Osteoporosis Foundation urges that people "think of your bones as a savings account. There is only as much bone mass in your account as you deposit."

In fact, osteoporosis is increasingly being viewed as a pediatric problem. According to Dr. Anne-Lise Carrié Fässler, an osteoporosis researcher in Switzerland, "Osteoporosis has long been considered a disease of the elderly; however, there is now a general agreement that predisposition begins in childhood and adolescence. Thus, rational approaches to prevention of the disease should be started during childhood and adolescence."

## Prevention

Building strong bones—especially before the age of 35—and then reducing bone loss in later years are the best strategies for preventing osteoporosis. Several risk factors predict those who should be most concerned about prevention of osteoporosis:

- **Age.** The older an individual, the greater the risk of osteoporosis, with most experiencing loss of bone mass starting in the fifth decade.
- **Gender.** Women are at greater risk for developing osteoporosis than men (four to one); they generally start with a lower peak bone mass and experience an accelerated loss following menopause.
- **Race.** Caucasian and Asian women are more likely to develop osteoporosis.
- **Bone structure and body weight.** Small-boned and thin women are at greater risk.
- **Menopause/menstrual history.** Normal or early menopause (brought about naturally or because of surgery) increases osteoporosis risk. In addition, women who stop menstruating before menopause because of conditions such as anorexia or bulimia, or

because of excessive physical exercise, may also lose bone tissue and develop osteoporosis.

- **Lifestyle.** With smoking, drinking too much alcohol, drinking more than two cups of coffee a day (when combined with a low calcium intake), consuming an inadequate amount of calcium, or getting little or no weight-bearing exercise, the chances of developing osteoporosis increase. A high caffeine intake (from any source including coffee, tea, and other beverages), a high protein intake from meat, fish, and eggs, and a high salt intake accelerate the loss of calcium in the urine, increasing the risk of bone fracture.

- **Medications and disease.** Osteoporosis is associated with certain medications (e.g., cortisone-like drugs, steroids, thyroid hormone, long-acting sedatives) and is a recognized complication of a number of medical conditions, including endocrine disorders (having an overactive thyroid), rheumatoid arthritis, chronic liver disease, and immobilization (e.g., prolonged bed rest).

- **Family history.** Susceptibility to fracture may be in part hereditary. Young women whose mothers have histories of vertebral fractures also seem to have reduced bone mass. Some researchers have estimated that 60 to 80 percent of bone mass is genetically determined.

Several tests can safely and accurately measure bone density. The newest, most accurate version uses a technology called DEXA—dual-energy X-ray absorptiometry. During the painless 15-minute scan, a low-dose, focused beam of radiation creates images of the hip and spine. A computer then calculates how dense the bones are as compared with those of healthy young adults and those of average people the same age. The cost is between $150 and $250. Most experts recommend against routine screening and suggest that DEXA measurements be reserved for high-risk individuals because of the high cost and limited testing resources. Osteoporosis is defined as a drop in bone density of 30 percent or more below the average bone density of healthy people in their 30s.

There is no cure for osteoporosis, but the National Osteoporosis Foundation does recommend several steps for slowing its progress:

- Diet
- Estrogen and other medications
- Exercise

According to an expert panel convened by the National Institutes of Health (NIH) in 1994, the optimal calcium intake to facilitate peak bone mass is 800 to 1,200 milligrams per day for older children, 1,200 to 1,500 milligrams per day for adolescents and young adults (ages 11 to 24 years), 1,000 milligrams per day for adult men and women, and 1,500 milligrams per day for elderly people and for women more than 50 years of age who are not on estrogens.

According to the NIH panel "The preferred source of calcium is through calcium-rich foods such as dairy products. Calcium-fortified foods and calcium supplements are other means by which optimal calcium intake can be reached in those who cannot meet this need by ingesting conventional foods."

There is growing evidence that when calcium intake is appropriate throughout life, a greater bone mass is developed in early adulthood, decreasing the risk of age-related bone loss. When calcium intake is too low (probably below 400 to 500 milligrams per day), peak bone mass may be below optimal levels. Too much caffeine, protein, and salt increase calcium loss in the urine.

Can calcium supplementation decrease bone loss after menopause? Several studies suggest yes, especially when combined with vitamin D and given to postmenopausal women with low calcium intakes.

Currently available medications include these:

• **Estrogen replacement therapy.** Estrogen has a direct and positive influence on bone cells. Following the loss of estrogen with menopause, bone loss is accelerated. A third to half of all bone loss in women is related to menopause. Since estrogen is so important for maintaining bone in women, physicians often prescribe estrogen replacement therapy for women at menopause. Estrogen replacement therapy is the only way to protect bone during the years of rapid bone loss immediately following menopause.

According to Dr. Lawrence Riggs of the Mayo Clinic, "If begun soon after the menopause, estrogen therapy prevents the early phase of bone loss, and decreases the incidence of fractures by about 50 percent." When started later in life, estrogen is also effective in preventing hip fractures. Other health benefits of using estrogen replacement therapy include decreased risk of coronary heart disease (risk drops in half), relief from hot flashes and other unpleasant symptoms of menopause, and decreased risk of colon cancer. Postmenopausal estrogen use has not been associated with weight gain (a fear that has caused many women to avoid it).

Taking estrogen alone does increase the risk of uterine cancer, but when synthetic progesterone is combined with the estrogen, the risk is eliminated. Although evidence is conflicting, there may be a small increase in risk of breast cancer after 15 years of hormone therapy. New evidence suggests that a high bone mineral density predicts the risk of breast cancer in older women, implying that long-term exposure to estrogen is an important risk factor for breast cancer. These concerns over estrogen have increased interest in the use of other medications for preventing and treating osteoporosis.

• **Calcitonin.** For men and women who already have osteoporosis, physicians will often prescribe the hormone calcitonin. It is also a treatment for women who cannot or choose not to take estrogen. Calcitonin is a naturally occurring hormone involved in calcium regulation and bone metabolism. Calcitonin safely prevents further bone loss by slowing bone removal and has been reported to provide relief from the pain associated with osteoporosis. An injectable form has been available for several years, but in 1995 the Food and Drug Administration approved a more user-friendly nasal spray (marketed as Miacalcin by Sandoz Pharmaceuticals Corp.).

• **Bisphosphonates.** These are compounds that inhibit bone breakdown and slow bone removal. They have been shown to increase bone density and decrease the risk of fractures. Alendronate sodium, marketed as Fosamax by Merck & Co., was approved by the Food and Drug Administration in 1995 for treating osteoporosis in postmenopausal women. Research by Dr. Dennis Black of the University of California, San Francisco, showed that Fosamax decreased the number of hip fractures by 51 percent over a three-year period among women with osteoporosis. This drug has few side effects when used properly. Serious irritations to the esophagus (the portion of the food tract between the throat and stomach) have been linked in some reports to taking Fosamax with very little water (six to eight ounces of water should be used to help wash the drug down to the stomach). Experts recommend taking Fosamax first thing in the morning with a full glass of water and avoiding lying down or consuming anything except water for at least 30 minutes afterward.

## EXERCISE-HEALTH CONNECTION

It is well known that humans lose bone mass rapidly when gravitational or muscle forces on the legs are decreased or become absent as in weightlessness, bed rest, or spinal cord injury. Healthy individuals who undergo complete bed rest for 4 to 36 weeks can lose an average of 1 percent bone mineral content per week, while astronauts in a gravity-free environment can lose bone at a monthly rate as high as 1 to 4 percent depending on the type of bone.

The National Aeronautics and Space Administration (NASA) realizes that long-term space travel by the human race will not be possible unless gravity can be simulated on board the spacecraft, protecting the skeleton. As Dr. Frank Sulzman of the NASA Space Medicine Branch has emphasized, "Our job is not only to make sure astronauts can function adequately in space, but also that they can function on their return to earth."

When force or stress is applied to a bone, the bone bends. This sets up a cascade of events that stimulate cells to strengthen the bone. The bone can adapt to stress or the lack of it by forming or losing mass. For the bone to become bigger and more dense, the stress must be above and beyond normal levels.

---

### Which is the best sporting activity I can undertake to reduce my risk of getting osteoporosis?

Many researchers have shown that athletes have a greater bone density than sedentary controls. Activities such as team sports, running, and racket sports, in which the weight of the body is borne by the feet and legs during vigorous movements, are more effective in maintaining density of the leg and spinal bones than nonweight-bearing activities such as bicycling and swimming.

---

The bone will continue to grow and adapt until it is restructured to handle the new imposed stress. This is one reason why total body weight has been found to be directly related to bone mineral density, with the heaviest people having the greatest bone density. In fact, one of the few benefits of being overweight is having unusually strong bones.

Figure 7.2 shows the results of an interesting study of female athletes and sedentary controls. Notice that volleyball and basketball athletes who engaged in jumping and short bursts of powerful leg movements had the greatest spine bone mineral density. Swimmers, who exercised in the near-weightless environment of water, had a bone density little different from that measured in the sedentary control subjects. Other studies have shown that athletes with the greatest bone mineral masses are weight lifters; next come athletes throwing the shot put and discus, then runners, soccer players, and finally swimmers.

Some researchers feel that differences in bone density between athletes and nonathletes may be due to factors of heredity and self-selection. In other words, people who do well in sport competition tend to have strong, dense bones to begin with. Although this may be true to a certain extent, studies comparing the active and inactive arms of tennis players, for example, show differences in bone density (i.e., the active

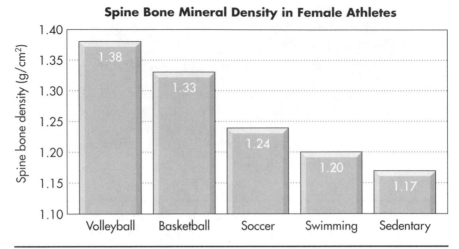

**FIGURE 7.2**    Athletes engaging in high impact, weight-bearing exercise have the greatest bone density.

arms of tennis players have stronger bones than the inactive arms). This suggests that bones adapt to the exercise stresses imposed directly upon them.

Among female athletes (especially runners and other endurance athletes) who lose their menstrual periods (called amenorrhea), bone mineral density typically decreases. The loss in bone density occurs even though they engage in vigorous endurance exercise. However, recent research with amenorrheic female gymnasts has shown that the extremely high stress on their skeletons from tumbling and dismount landings can actually override the negative effects of low reproductive hormones.

Thus it appears that in some cases, if the exercise stress is high enough, the bone will strengthen regardless of the poor hormonal environment. Dr. Snow cautions, however, that "there is no basis for the claim that exercise is superior to estrogen as a deterrent to bone loss." Female endurance athletes who are amenorrheic should attempt to regain their menstrual period or use estrogen therapy to avoid early osteoporosis. Running is an insufficient stimulus to counteract the loss of estrogen that occurs with amenorrhea, and few women are willing to undergo the intense gymnastic-like exercise that is necessary to protect bone mass under these conditions.

As emphasized by the President's Council on Physical Fitness and Sports, "The foundation for bone health begins early in life. Physical activity that places a load on the bones is essential throughout childhood and the adolescent years."

## How old is too old to benefit from exercise as a way to stop osteoporosis?

Some researchers feel that young bone is more responsive to exercise stress than old bone. Given that approximately 60 percent of the final skeleton is built during adolescence, vigorous physical exercise during childhood and adolescence is probably more important than at any other time in life.

Children who engage in sports that produce much stress on the skeleton (e.g., running, gymnastics, and dance) have been found to have greater bone density than children who are swimmers or who engage in no sports at all. Researchers in Sweden have shown that adolescents who have stronger muscles through regular exercise also have denser bones. This is an important finding, because the development of strong and dense bones early in life should translate to less osteoporosis in old age.

Among older women, researchers have found that a history of lifelong physical activity relates to a greater bone mineral mass, and very importantly, a lowered risk of hip fracture. Several studies have now shown that muscle strength is an important predictor of strong and dense bones among older adults. Typically, as people age, both bone density and muscular strength decrease, as shown in figure 7.3. Dr.

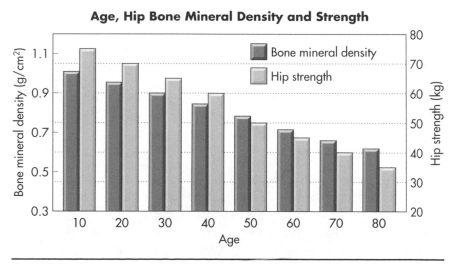

**FIGURE 7.3**  As women age, bone mineral density of the hip joint decreases in proportion to strength.

Christine Snow of the Bone Research Laboratory, Oregon State University, has shown that muscular strength has an important influence on bone mineral density at all sites among women. In other words, if women maintain good muscle strength through intensive exercise, bone density should be better preserved even into old age.

---

### I'm taking estrogen to prevent bone loss. If I exercise, can I stop taking the estrogen?

No. Most experts recommend that a multifaceted approach to treatment of osteoporosis be pursued, with exercise seen as one of several essential components.

---

According to the National Osteoporosis Foundation, "Exercise alone cannot prevent or cure osteoporosis." The American College of Sports Medicine (ACSM) adds that although "weight-bearing physical activity is essential for the normal development and maintenance of a healthy skeleton . . . exercise cannot be recommended as a substitute for hormone replacement therapy at the time of menopause." In other words, osteoporosis prevention and treatment demand a multifaceted approach.

Exercise has not received enthusiastic support by some authorities as an effective way to treat osteoporosis. For example, the 1988 Surgeon General's report on nutrition and health was reserved in its endorsement, concluding that "until better information becomes available, three to four hours of weight-bearing exercise per week is potentially beneficial to the skeleton and could represent a safe, low-cost method for maintaining bone mass."

Since 1988, volumes of information have been published on exercise and osteoporosis. In reviewing this information, the ACSM has established that five principles should be considered in evaluating the success of an exercise program for preventing or treating osteoporosis:

- **Principle of specificity.** If the leg bones are stressed by running and jumping, the arm bones will not benefit unless they too are stressed with specific exercises (e.g., weight lifting).
- **Principle of overload.** For a bone to improve its density and strength, the exercise stress must exceed normal levels.
- **Principle of reversibility.** The positive effect of an exercise program on the skeleton will be lost if the program is stopped.

- **Principle of initial values.** People with the lowest levels of bone density and strength will experience more improvement from an exercise program than those with normal or above-normal bone density.
- **Principle of diminishing returns.** Each person has an individual genetic ceiling that limits the gains in bone mass. As this ceiling is approached, gains in bone mass will slow and plateau.

---

### What type of exercise program is most effective in treating osteoporosis?

It is becoming increasingly apparent that physical activities such as walking or swimming do not place enough stress on the bones to improve their strength. Results from several studies investigating the effect of walking show that this activity, commonly recommended for postmenopausal women, does not prevent bone loss. Other studies that have included physical activities of higher intensity and weight lifting have shown a more positive effect on the skeleton.

---

In a one-year study of 39 postmenopausal women, subjects engaged in intensive weight training for 45 minutes, two times a week. Compared to control subjects, they improved their strength and muscle mass as well as their bone mineral density. This study shows the value of intensive resistance training in protecting the skeleton. According to Dr. Miriam Nelson of Tufts University, who headed up the study, "All of these outcomes may mediate a reduction of the risk for future osteoporotic fractures."

Dr. Richard Prince of the University of Western Australia studied 120 postmenopausal women and showed that aerobic exercise alone (without weight training) had no effect on density of the forearm bone (a bone that is not stressed during most aerobic activities). As shown in figure 7.4, at first glance it would appear that estrogen when combined with exercise had a positive effect on forearm bone density. However, a closer review of the results shows that the improvement in forearm bone density was due to estrogen. This study shows the value of estrogen therapy in relation to bone density, as well as the low value of exercise if it is not intensive and not directed to the bone being measured.

In another one-year study of postmenopausal women (32 women, 60 to 72 years of age), Dr. Wendy Kohrt of the Washington University

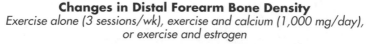

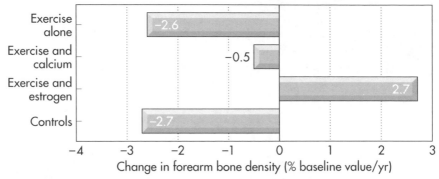

FIGURE 7.4  Exercise alone has little effect on forearm bone density compared to estrogen.

School of Medicine in St. Louis measured the influence of vigorous weight-bearing exercise on spinal bone mineral density. The women walked and jogged and climbed stairs vigorously for 50 minutes a session, three to four times a week. Exercise and estrogen therapy together had the greatest effect on lumbar bone density, with about one-third of the improvement due to exercise. Concludes Dr. Kohrt, "The results of this study suggest that the efficacy of estrogen therapy would be enhanced by combining it with weight-bearing exercise."

One of the chief benefits of regular exercise by elderly persons is a decrease in the risk of falling. Falls and the resulting injuries are among the most serious and common medical problems encountered by those who are elderly. Each year, about 3 in 10 elderly individuals sustain a fall, with 10 to 15 percent of falls resulting in serious injuries such as hip fractures.

The ACSM in its position statement on osteoporosis and exercise has urged that "the optimal program for older women would include activities that improve strength, flexibility, and coordination that may indirectly, but effectively, decrease the incidence of osteoporotic fractures by lessening the likelihood of falling."

Researchers led by Dr. Michael Province of the Washington University School of Medicine studied about 2,300 elderly individuals in six different states and showed that treatments including exercise reduced the risk of falls. In other words, regular weight-bearing and resistance exercise has a twofold benefit for elderly people—an improvement in bone mineral density and a reduced likelihood of falling.

# REFERENCES

American College of Sports Medicine. (1995). ACSM position stand on osteoporosis and exercise. *Medicine and Science in Sports and Exercise, 27,* i-vii.

Bailey, D.A., Faulkner, R.A., & McKay, H.A. (1996). Growth, physical activity, and bone mineral acquisition. In J.O. Holloszy (Ed.), *Exercise and Sports Science Review, 24,* 233-263.

Bloomfield, S.A. (1997). Changes in musculoskeletal structure and function with prolonged bed rest. *Medicine and Science in Sports and Exercise, 29,* 197-206.

Cauley, J.A., Lucas, L.L., Kuller, L.H., Vogt, M.T., Browner, W.S., & Cummings, S.R. (1996). Bone mineral density and risk of breast cancer in older women: The study of osteoporotic fractures. *Journal of the American Medical Association, 276,* 1404-1408.

Dook, J.E., James, C., Henderson, N.K., & Price, R.I. (1997). Exercise and bone mineral density in mature female athletes. *Medicine and Science in Sports and Exercise, 29,* 291-296.

Farley, D. (1996, April). New ways to heal broken bones. *FDA Consumer,* 14-18.

Fässler, A.L., & Bonjour, J.P. (1995). Osteoporosis as a pediatric problem. *Pediatric Clinics of North America, 42,* 811-824.

Kohrt, W.M., Snead, D.B., Slatopolsky, E., & Birge, S.J. (1995). Additive effects of weight-bearing exercise and estrogen on bone mineral density in older women. *Journal of Bone and Mineral Research, 10,* 1303-1311.

Lee, E.J., Long, K.A., Risser, W.L., Poindexter, H.B.W., Gibbons, W.E., & Goldzieher, J. (1995). Variations in bone status of contralateral and regional sites in young athletic women. *Medicine and Science in Sports and Exercise, 27,* 1354-1361.

Meyer, H.E., Pedersen, J.I., Løken, E.B., & Tverdal, A. (1997). Dietary factors and the incidence of hip fracture in middle-aged Norwegians. *American Journal of Epidemiology, 145,* 117-123.

Nelson, M.E., Fiatarone, M.A., Morganti, C.M., Trice, I., Greenberg, R.A., & Evans, W.J. (1994). Effects of high-intensity strength training on multiple risk factors for osteoporotic fractures: A randomized controlled trial. *Journal of the American Medical Association, 272,* 1909-1914.

NIH Consensus Development Panel on Optimal Calcium Intake. (1994). Optimal calcium intake. *Journal of the American Medical Association, 272,* 1942-1948.

Province, M.A., Hadley, E.C., Hornbrook, M.C., et al. (1995). The effects of exercise on falls in elderly patients: A preplanned meta-analysis of the FICSIT Trials. *Journal of the American Medical Association, 273,* 1341-1347.

Riggs, B.L., & Melton, L.J. (1992). The prevention and treatment of osteoporosis. *New England Journal of Medicine, 327,* 620-627.

Schneider, D.L., Barrett-Connor, E.L., & Morton, D.J. (1997). Timing of postmenopausal estrogen for optimal bone mineral density. The Rancho Bernardo Study. *Journal of the American Medical Association, 277,* 543-547.

Snow, C.M. (1996). Exercise and bone mass in young and premenopausal women. *Bone, 18* (Suppl.), 51S-55S.

U.S. Preventive Services Task Force. (1996). *Guide to clinical preventive services* (2nd ed.). Alexandria, VA: International Medical.

# Chapter 8

# ARTHRITIS

Available data may be interpreted to suggest that reasonable recreational exercise—carried out within limits of comfort,
putting joints through normal motions, and without
underlying joint abnormality—need not inevitably
lead to joint injury, even over many years.

**Dr. Richard Panush, Department of Medicine, New Jersey Medical School**

Arthritis as a disease dates to antiquity. Bones of the Java Ape Man and the mummies of Egypt show signs of arthritic damage. The Roman emperor Diocletian exempted citizens with severe arthritis from paying taxes, no doubt feeling that the disease itself can be taxing enough.

## Prevalence

Arthritis and other rheumatic conditions are among the most prevalent chronic conditions in the United States, affecting an estimated 40 million persons in 1995 (one in seven) and a projected 60 million by 2020, according to the Centers for Disease Control and Prevention.

Women are affected by arthritis more than men; nearly two-thirds of people with arthritis are women. Arthritis is the number-one cause of disability in America. It limits everyday activities such as dressing, climbing stairs, getting in and out of bed, or walking, for about seven million Americans.

## Pathogenesis

Arthritis, meaning joint inflammation, is a general term that includes over 100 kinds of rheumatic diseases. Rheumatic diseases are those affecting joints, muscles, and connective tissue, which make up or support various structures of the body. Arthritis is usually chronic, meaning that it lasts a lifetime. The early warning signs of arthritis include pain, swelling, and limited movement that lasts for more than two weeks.

The most common type of arthritis is osteoarthritis, affecting more than 16 million Americans and about half of those 65 years of age and older. Although this degenerative joint disease is common among elderly people, it may appear decades earlier. Osteoarthritis begins when joint cartilage breaks down, sometimes eroding entirely to leave a bone-on-bone joint. Any joint can be affected, but occurrence is most common in the feet, knees, hips, and fingers.

In a normal joint, where two bones meet, the ends are coated with cartilage, a smooth, slippery cushion that protects the bone and reduces friction during movement. In osteoarthritis, cartilage breaks down and the bones rub together. The joint then loses shape, bone ends thicken, and spurs (bony growths) develop (see figure 8.1).

Osteoarthritis is not fatal, but it is incurable, with few effective treatments. Symptoms of pain and stiffness can persist for long periods of time, leading to difficulty in walking, stair climbing, rising from a chair, transferring in and out of a car, and lifting and carrying, all of which are necessary to maintain independence and a good quality of life.

Second most common is rheumatoid arthritis, an autoimmune disease that affects 2.5 million Americans, three times more women than men. It can strike at any age, but usually appears between ages 20 and 50. Rheumatoid arthritis starts slowly over several weeks to months. The small joints of the hands and the knee joint are most commonly affected, but rheumatoid arthritis can affect most joints of the body. In general, it is frequently related to severe complications and decline in ability to function, with most patients dying 10 to 15 years earlier than those who are do not have the disease.

Many joints of the body have a tough capsule lined with a synovial membrane that seals the joint and provides a lubricating fluid. In rheumatoid arthritis, inflammation begins in the synovial lining of the joint and can spread to the entire joint. The inflamed joint lining leads to damage of the bone and cartilage. The space between joints diminishes, and the joint loses shape and alignment. Highly variable (some people with this form of arthritis become bedridden, while others can run marathons) and difficult to control, the disease can severely deform joints.

Other common types of arthritis include gout (a metabolic disorder leading to high uric acid and crystal formation in joints), ankylosing spondylitis (inflammatory disease of the spine), juvenile arthritis (involving 200,000 American children), psoriatic arthritis (affecting about

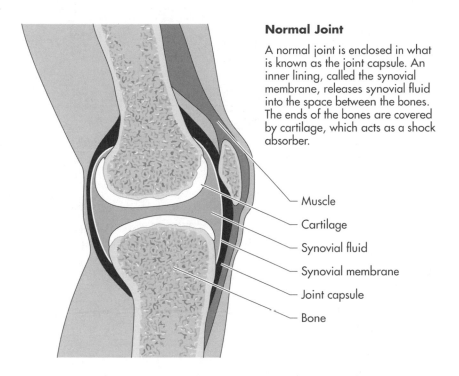

### Normal Joint

A normal joint is enclosed in what is known as the joint capsule. An inner lining, called the synovial membrane, releases synovial fluid into the space between the bones. The ends of the bones are covered by cartilage, which acts as a shock absorber.

Muscle

Cartilage

Synovial fluid

Synovial membrane

Joint capsule

Bone

### Osteoarthritis Joint

In a joint with osteoarthritis, cartilage breaks down and causes bones to rub together. Bone ends thicken and form painful growths called spurs.

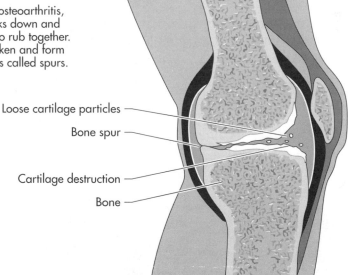

Loose cartilage particles

Bone spur

Cartilage destruction

Bone

**FIGURE 8.1**   The development of osteoarthritis.

5 percent of people with psoriasis, a chronic skin disease), and systemic lupus erythematosus (symptoms usually appearing in women of child-bearing age).

## Treatment

With so many kinds of arthritis, and the unpredictable nature of this disease, diagnosis and treatment can be troublesome. According to the Arthritis Foundation, many things can be done to reduce the impact of arthritis on everyday life. The key is early diagnosis and a treatment plan tailored to the needs of each patient.

Therapy of arthritis has four major goals: easing pain, decreasing painful inflammation, improving function, and lessening joint damage. Most treatment programs include a combination of patient education, medication, exercise, rest, use of heat and cold, joint-protection techniques, and sometimes surgery (for example, total hip replacement surgery).

According to the American College of Rheumatology guidelines, treatment should include the following:

- **Lifestyle changes**—exercise to strengthen muscles, weight loss to reduce stress on joints, and assistive devices such as canes and wall bars when needed

- **Pain management**—physical therapy, acetaminophen as first-line therapy, and prescription drugs or surgery for more severe pain

- **Patient education**—informing patients about the disease and providing tools to help overcome pain and help them adjust to their situation

Arthritis will wax and wane on its own. A worsening or reappearance of the disease is called a flare. This can be followed by a remission period that brings welcome relief. The normal up-and-down nature of this painful, incurable disease has led to widespread fraud and quackery. People with arthritis spend nearly a billion dollars a year on unproven remedies, largely diets and supplements, according to the Food and Drug Administration (FDA).

Arthritis patients have been lured by an astounding array of quack devices, including copper or magnetic bracelets, "electronic" mechanisms, vibrating chairs, pressurized enema devices, snake venom, and countless nutritional supplements including cod liver oil, alfalfa, poke-berries, vinegar, iodine, and kelp. According to the FDA, while some of these remedies seem harmless, they can become hurtful if they cause people to abandon conventional therapy.

The FDA also cautions that diet has little to do with arthritis. Gout is the only rheumatic disease known to be helped by avoidance of certain foods. Regarding diet, the American College of Rheumatology advises that "until more data are available, patients should continue to follow balanced and healthy diets, be skeptical of 'miraculous' claims and avoid elimination diets and fad nutritional practices."

Overweight persons are at high risk of osteoarthritis in the knee, hips, and hands. For example, the risk of developing osteoarthritis of the knee is 7 to 10 times greater for the heaviest Americans (those in the upper 20 percent of body weight) than for those of normal weight. Weight control is an important concern for people with arthritis. Keeping close to ideal weight helps decrease the pressure on the knees and hips. In a study supported by the Arthritis Foundation, researchers found that overweight, middle-aged and older women could significantly lower their risk for developing osteoarthritis of the knee by losing weight. "By losing weight or avoiding excessive weight gain, you can reduce the amount of pain and limitations from osteoarthritis if you have the disease, and you can reduce your chances of ever developing the condition if you don't yet have it," concludes Dr. Doyt Conn, medical editor for *Arthritis Today*.

Many different kinds of drugs are used to treat arthritis. Anti-inflammatory agents generally work by slowing the body's production of prostaglandins, substances that play a role in inflammation. The most familiar anti-inflammatory agent is aspirin, often a good arthritis treatment. Acetaminophen is recommended as a first-line therapy, at doses up to 4,000 milligrams a day.

More than a dozen nonsteroidal anti-inflammatory drugs (NSAIDs) are available, most by prescription only, for fighting pain and inflammation. The FDA has approved three NSAIDs for over-the-counter marketing: ibuprofen (marketed as Advil, Nuprin, Motrin, and others), naproxen sodium (sold as Aleve), and ketoprofen (marketed as Actron and Orudis). The most potent anti-inflammatories are corticosteroids.

Disease-modifying drugs are also prescribed by physicians to slow rheumatoid arthritis. These drugs are now used early in the course of the illness to retard disease advancement. Gold salts, penicillamine, methotrexate, hydroxychloroquine, sulfasalazine, and other powerful drugs, often employed in combination, are used to help suppress the immune system.

## EXERCISE-HEALTH CONNECTION

In the past, physicians often advised arthritis patients to rest and avoid exercise. Rest remains important, especially during flares. But inactivity can lead to weak muscles, stiff joints, reduced joint range of motion, and decreased energy and vitality. Now rheumatologists routinely advise a balance of physical activity and rest, individualized to meet special patient needs.

---

### Can I exercise if I have arthritis?

A comprehensive physical fitness program designed to improve joint range of motion and flexibility, muscular strength and endurance, and aerobic endurance, and individualized to the patient's special needs and goals, is recommended.

---

Many studies have shown that people with arthritis have weaker muscles, less joint flexibility and range of motion, and lower aerobic capacity than those without arthritis. In addition, individuals with arthritis have been found to be at higher risk for several other chronic diseases including coronary heart disease, diabetes mellitus, and osteoporosis.

Thus it makes sense that a well-rounded physical fitness program may benefit those who have arthritis. As Dr. Walter Ettinger of the Bowman Gray School of Medicine in North Carolina has emphasized, "A substantial portion of the disability from arthritis is due to loss of physical capacity that is in part correctable through exercise training."

Individuals with arthritis will often respond to their pain by limiting physical activity. Over time, this leads to loss of muscle strength and endurance, further weakening the joints, thus setting up a vicious cycle that accelerates arthritis.

According to most experts, there are three objectives of exercise for patients with arthritis:

- Preserving or restoring range of motion and flexibility around each affected joint
- Increasing muscle strength and endurance to enhance joint stability
- Increasing aerobic conditioning to improve psychological mood state and decrease risk of disease

As depicted in figure 8.2, the exercise program should be organized according to the "Exercise Pyramid," with exercises to develop joint range of motion and flexibility providing the foundation. "Prior to

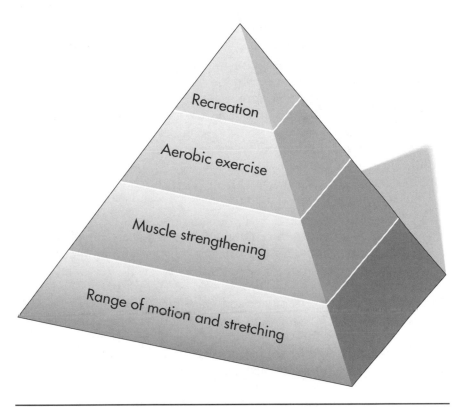

FIGURE 8.2   Exercise pyramid for patients with arthritis.

initiating an exercise program, each patient should have an extensive evaluation to assess the severity and extent of joint involvement, presence of systemic involvement, overall functional capacity, and presence of other medical conditions that may interfere with exercise," cautions Dr. Douglas Hoffman of the Department of Sports Medicine, Physicians Plus Medical Group, Middleton, Wisconsin.

• **Range of motion and stretching exercises:** Joints are designed for movement, and they require motion to stay healthy. Maintaining joint mobility is very important for all patients with arthritis. Loss of joint range of motion results in a tightening of surrounding tendons, muscles, and other tissues. Acutely inflamed joints should be put through gentle range-of-motion exercises several times per day with the assistance of a therapist or trained family member. Overzealous stretching or improper technique can have harmful effects on a joint, especially if it is inflamed or is unstable. Utilizing a trained therapist to initially monitor and teach the patient proper technique is recommended. Once the joints become less inflamed, the patient can gradually build up to several sets of 10 repetitions daily of stretching and range-of-motion exercises.

• **Muscle strengthening:** Both isometric (muscle contraction without movement) and isotonic (muscle contraction with joint movement) strengthening exercises are recommended. Isometric exercises can build muscle strength without adverse effects on an acutely inflamed joint. Isotonic exercises (e.g., weight lifting, calisthenics, leg movement during bicycling) allow the joint to move through a limited or full range of motion while the muscle is contracting. This type of exercise is recommended when pain and joint inflammation have been controlled and sufficient strength has been achieved through isometric exercise.

• **Aerobic exercise:** In the past, the treatment of arthritis has often excluded aerobic exercise for fear of increasing joint inflammation and accelerating the disease process. Aerobic exercise, however, has been demonstrated to be a safe and effective treatment for patients who are not in acute flares. Low-impact activities such as swimming, water aerobics, walking, bicycling, low-impact dance aerobics, and rowing can improve aerobic fitness without negatively affecting arthritis. Patients should start with 10 to 15 minutes of aerobic activity every other day, gradually progressing toward near-daily activity of 30 to 45 minutes' duration at a moderate to somewhat hard intensity. Each aerobic session should begin and end with range-of-motion exercises.

• **Recreational exercise:** Golfing, gardening, hiking on gentle terrain, and other hobbies requiring physical activity are examples of activities that patients with arthritis commonly find enjoyable. Many organizations, including the Arthritis Foundation and PACE (People with Arthritis Can Exercise), offer aquatic exercise classes or other group activities. Patients may experience improvements in both fitness and psychological mood state as they engage in group recreational activities. The Arthritis Foundation information line is 800-283-7800.

---

### Can regular exercise keep my arthritis from getting worse?

Joint range-of-motion exercises for flexibility, strengthening exercises, and aerobic conditioning exercises have been shown in most studies to be safe and effective in improving physical fitness for patients with osteoarthritis or rheumatoid arthritis. Less clear are the therapeutic benefits of exercise, with most studies reporting that arthritis is not improved or worsened because of exercise training.

There are many potential benefits of exercise for the individual with arthritis:

- Improvement in joint function and range of motion
- Increase in muscular strength and aerobic fitness to enhance daily activities of living
- Elevation of psychological mood state
- Decrease in loss of bone mass
- Decrease in risk of heart disease, diabetes, hypertension, and other chronic diseases

Can regular exercise improve, retard the progression, or even cure arthritis? Most researchers who have studied this question now answer no. While exercise for people with arthritis is important for all the reasons just listed, investigators have typically found that exercise training does not improve arthritis but that it does not worsen the disease process either. In other words, exercise does not affect the underlying disease state in people with arthritis one way or the other, but does improve many other areas of importance to life quality.

Dr. Pamela Kovar of Columbia University, for example, randomly divided 102 patients with osteoarthritis of the knee into walking and control groups. Those in the walking group walked up to 30 minutes, three times a week, for eight weeks. As shown in figure 8.3, the walkers

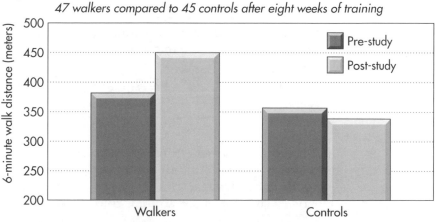

**Supervised Fitness Walking in Patients With Osteoarthritis of the Knee**
*47 walkers compared to 45 controls after eight weeks of training*

FIGURE 8.3    Eight weeks walking (3 times/week, 90 minutes/session) improved 6-minute walking performance.

experienced a strong increase in their performance during a six-minute walking test, an effect, says Dr. Kovar, "that was achieved without exacerbating pain or triggering flares." In other words, those with osteoarthritis became fitter with the exercise program, but their disease was not reversed.

Dr. Eric Coleman of the University of Washington in Seattle divided elderly subjects with a history of mild to moderate arthritis into four groups: strength training (two sets and 10 repetitions of eight different weight machine exercises, three days a week), stationary cycle training (35 minutes at 60 to 75 percent intensity, three days a week), both strength and cycle training, and controls. After six months of training, strength improved significantly in all exercise groups, but especially in those who worked out on the weight machines. Joint pain symptoms did not improve or worsen in any group. "In this study, we found no evidence that well regulated exercise produces or exacerbates joint pain in healthy community-dwelling older adults with mild to moderate joint symptoms," concluded Dr. Coleman.

Other researchers have come to the same conclusion: patients with arthritis are trainable (i.e., they can get stronger and more aerobically fit), and the exercise can be done safely without detrimental effects on the joints. However, as emphasized by Dr. Troels Hansen of Herlev University Hospital in Denmark, who measured the influence of exercise training in 75 patients with rheumatoid arthritis over a two-year period, "The results showed no effect of training on the disease activity or on the progression of the disease."

---

### I've played sports and exercised for years. Has that increased my chances of getting arthritis?

Most experts feel that athletic participation does not increase the risk of osteoarthritis unless the participant has an underlying joint abnormality or major injury.

---

Some clinicians have defined osteoarthritis as a "wear and tear" disease. Individuals who exercise faithfully may be sacrificing their joints for the health of their heart, some critics assert.

Several important risk factors for osteoarthritis include the following:

- **Increasing age:** By 75 years of age, 85 percent of people have evidence of osteoarthritis.

- **Joint malalignment:** If the joint is not aligned properly, a smaller contact area may create stresses that exceed the shock-absorbing capabilities of the joint.
- **Obesity:** Several studies have suggested that obesity increases the risk for osteoarthritis.
- **Repetitive impact to the joint:** In some sports, the joints are subjected to high-impact and unnatural forces that may increase the risk for osteoarthritis later in life. This risk factor, however, is the topic of considerable debate among researchers. Some animal studies have suggested that animals that have been trained intensely for long time periods have more osteoarthritis. For example, the Husky breed of dogs has increased hip and shoulder arthritis from pulling sleds, while racehorses and workhorses can develop arthritis in their forelegs and hind legs, respectively.

Together, these risk factors and animal studies appear to suggest that osteoarthritis is a wear-and-tear disease. Most experts feel, however, that evidence to confirm this perception in humans is lacking.

Earlier studies had suggested that repetitive trauma to joints during work may lead to arthritis. For example, some studies reported increased osteoarthritis in the elbows and knees of miners, in the shoulders and elbows of pneumatic drill operators, in the hands of cotton workers and diamond cutters, and in the spines of dock workers. However, as Dr. Richard Panush of the Department of Medicine, New Jersey Medical School, has cautioned, "Not all of these studies were carried out to contemporary standards, nor have they been confirmed."

Is regular participation in sport and exercise associated with osteoarthritis? Many athletic endeavors place tremendous stress on joints. Baseball, football, basketball, gymnastics, soccer, wrestling, and ballet dancing have each been studied for their effect on osteoarthritis. There are many anecdotal reports of famous athletes developing arthritis. Los Angeles Dodger Sandy Koufax, for example, was forced to retire from pitching in 1966 because of an arthritic elbow.

Most experts, however, feel that participation in vigorous exercise and sport does not increase the risk of osteoarthritis unless the involved joint has some sort of abnormality or previous major injury. Normal joints are well designed to withstand the repetitive stress that comes with physical activity. But an injury to the joint alters its ability to handle exercise stress. Several studies of athletes with major knee injuries, for example, have shown that they are at increased risk of premature osteoarthritis.

Long-distance runners have been studied more than any other type of athlete because of the long-term and repetitive stress they experience to joints of their legs. During running, two and one-half to three times the body weight is transmitted to the lower limbs at heel strike. The stresses that the feet and ankles do not absorb are shifted to the knees, hips, and spine.

Despite the repetitive stress to their feet and legs, long-distance runners who train for many years do not appear to be at increased risk of osteoarthritis unless they have abnormal biomechanical problems or prior injuries in the hips, knees, or ankles. Most studies have shown, according to Dr. Nancy Lane of the Division of Rheumatology, University of California in San Francisco, "that long-duration high-mileage running need not be associated with premature degenerative joint disease in the lower extremities."

The injury rate among participants in many sports is quite high. Fortunately, most injuries appear to be limited, with no long-term consequences. If the injury leads to long-term joint instability, however, the risk for osteoarthritis climbs sharply. As summarized by Dr. Panush, "Available data may be interpreted to suggest that reasonable recreational exercise—carried out within limits of comfort, putting joints through normal motions, and without underlying joint abnormality—need not inevitably lead to joint injury, even over many years."

# REFERENCES

Coleman, E.A., Buchner, D.M., Cress, M.E., Chan, B.K.S., & de Lateur, B.J. (1996). The relationship of joint symptoms with exercise performance in older adults. *Journal of the American Geriatric Society, 44,* 14-21.

Ettinger, W.H., & Afable, R.F. (1994). Physical disability from knee osteoarthritis: The role of exercise as an intervention. *Medicine and Science in Sports and Exercise, 26,* 1435-1440.

Ettinger, W.H., Burns, R., Messier, S.P., Applegate, W., Rejeski, W.J., Morgan, T., Shumaker, S., Berry, M.J., O'Toole, M., Monu, J., & Craven, T. (1997). A randomized trial comparing aerobic exercise and resistance exercise with a health education program in older adults with knee osteoarthritis. The Fitness Arthritis and Seniors Trial (FAST). *Journal of the American Medical Association, 277,* 25-31.

Felson, D.T. (1996). Weight and osteoarthritis. *American Journal of Clinical Nutrition, 63* (Suppl.), 430S-432S.

Hochberg, M.C., Altman, R.D., & Brandt, K.D. (1995). Guidelines for the medical management of knee osteoarthritis. *Arthritis Rheumatology, 38,* 1541-1546.

Hoffman, D.F. (1993). Arthritis and exercise. *Primary Care, 20*, 895-910.

Häkkinen, A., Häkkinen, K., & Hannonen, P. (1994). *Scandanavian Journal of Rheumatology, 23*, 237-242.

Hanson, T.M., Hansen, G., Langgaard, A.M., & Rasmussen, J.O. (1993). Longterm physical training in rheumatoid arthritis. A randomized trial with different training programs and blinded observers. *Scandanavian Journal of Rheumatology, 22*, 107-112.

Kovar, P.A., Allegrante, J.P., MacKenzie, R., Peterson, M.G.E., Gutin, B., & Charlson, M.E. (1992). Supervised fitness walking in patients with osteoarthritis of the knee. *Annals of Internal Medicine, 116*, 529-534.

Lane, N.E., & Buckwalter, J.A. (1993). Exercise: A cause of osteoarthritis? *Rheumatic Disease Clinics of North America, 19*, 617-633.

Lyngberg, K.K., Harreby, M., Bentzen, H., Frost, B., & Danneskiold-Samsøe. (1994). Elderly rheumatoid arthritis patients on steroid treatment tolerate physical training without an increase in disease activity. *Archives of Physical Medicine and Rehabilitation, 75*, 1189-1195.

Panush, R.S. (1994). Physical activity, fitness, and osteoarthritis. In C. Bouchard, R.J. Shephard, & T. Stephens (Eds.), *Physical activity, fitness, and health: International proceedings and consensus statement* (pp. 712-722). Champaign, IL: Human Kinetics.

Rall, L.C., Meydani, S.N., Kehayias, J.J., Dawson-Hughes, B., & Roubenoff, R. (1996). The effect of progressive resistance training in rheumatoid arthritis. Increased strength without changes in energy balance or body composition. *Arthritis Rheumatology, 39*, 415-426.

Semble, E.L. (1995). Rheumatoid arthritis: New approaches for its evaluation and management. *Archives of Physical Medicine and Rehabilitation, 76*, 190-201.

Strange, C.J. (1996, March). Coping with arthritis in its many forms. *FDA Consumer*, 17-21.

Ytterberg, S.R., Mahowald, M.L., & Krug, H.E. (1994). Exercise for arthritis. *Baillière's Clinical Rheumatology, 8*, 161-189.

# Chapter 9

# LOW BACK PAIN

*Our controlled study of workers with acute low back pain suggests that avoiding bed rest and maintaining ordinary activity as tolerated lead to the most rapid recovery.*

**Dr. Antti Malmivaara, Finnish Institute of Occupational Health, Helsinki, Finland**

Joan Benoit Samuelson is regarded by many experts as the best American female long-distance runner in history, a record highlighted by her gold medal victory in the 1984 Olympic Marathon. Joan and her husband, Scott, have two children, born three and five years after Joan's Olympic experience. Throughout both pregnancies, Joan continued to train, running more than six miles a day. Following her first delivery, she returned to running too soon and developed pain in her lower back and hips. "Perhaps I did not give my lower back and pelvic ligaments a chance to return to their original function and position," Joan recalls. "In fact, this may have caused the slight misalignment in my hips that I have had ever since. Since the birth of my children, I've had problems with my lower back and hips."

## Prevalence

Low back pain levies a heavy toll upon modern men and women. At some point in their lives, 60 to 80 percent of all Americans and Europeans will experience a bout of low back pain that may range from a dull, annoying ache to intense and prolonged pain. After headaches, low back pain is the second most common ailment in the United States, topped only by colds and flus in time lost from work. Next to arthritis, low back pain is the most frequently reported disability.

A nationwide government survey revealed that back pain lasting for at least a week is reported by 18 percent of the working population each year. Of these people, about half attribute the cause of the back pain to a work-related activity or injury, with the proportion much higher among workers in farming, forestry, or fishing occupations. This problem is not unique to the civilian population; back pain accounts for at least 20 percent of all medical discharges from the U.S. Army.

Low back pain commonly affects people in their most productive years, resulting in a substantial economic cost to society. When all the costs connected with low back pain are added up—job absenteeism, medical and legal fees, social security disability payments, workers' compensation, long-term disability insurance—the bill to business, industry, and the government has been estimated to range from $16 to $50 billion per year.

Males and females appear to be affected equally, with most cases of low back pain occurring between the ages of 25 and 60 years with a peak at about 40 years of age. The first attack often occurs early in life, however, with up to one-third of adolescents reporting that they have experienced at least one bout of low back pain. A 25-year study of school children in Denmark showed that low back pain during the growth period is an important risk factor for low back pain later in life. Because of this, Dr. Mette Harreby of Copenhagen, who headed up the study, feels that "implementing preventive measures in schools may be very important."

Fortunately, most low back pain is self-limiting. Without treatment, 60 percent of people with back pain return to work within a week, and nearly 90 percent return within six weeks. A significant proportion (at least one-third) of those experiencing low back pain once have recurrent episodes. Pain remains for up to 5 to 10 percent of patients, creating a chronic condition. About 70 to 90 percent of the total costs related to back pain are borne by these patients.

## Pathology

Knowing a little about the spine and its parts makes it easier to understand why things can go wrong with the back, which is composed of 24 vertebrae, 23 disks, 31 pairs of spinal nerves, and 140 attaching muscles, plus a large number of ligaments and tendons (see figure 9.1). Although humans are born with 33 separate vertebrae (the bones that form the spine), by adulthood most have only 24. The 9 vertebrae at the base of the spine grow together; 5 form the sacrum, while the lowest 4 form the coccyx. There are 7 cervical vertebrae that support and provide movement for the head (C1 to C7), while 12 thoracic vertebrae join with and are supported by the ribs (T1 to T12). The 5 lumbar vertebrae (L1 to L5)

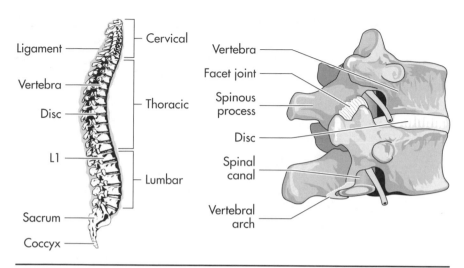

**FIGURE 9.1**   The anatomy of the spine and vertebra.

are most frequently involved in back pain because they carry most of the body's stress. Anatomically, the term "low back pain syndrome" is applied to pain experienced in the lumbosacral region (L1 to S1 vertebrae). The most commonly indicated site of low back pain is the L4-L5 lumbar segment.

## Prevention

Various risk factors for low back pain have been advanced. It is believed that many cases of low back pain are due to unusual stresses on the muscles and ligaments that support the spine of susceptible individuals. When the body is in poor shape, for example, weak spinal and abdominal muscles may be unable to support the spine properly during certain types of lifting or physical activities.

But even hardy occupational workers or athletes who exercise beyond their tolerance are susceptible. Rowers, triathletes, professional golfers and tennis players, wrestlers, and gymnasts, for example, have all been reported to have high rates of back injury. Jobs that involve bending and twisting, or lifting heavy objects repeatedly (especially when the loads are beyond a worker's strength), are a chief cause of low back pain.

Certain occupations, such as truck or bus driving, fire fighting, and nursing, are particularly hard on the back. The truck driver, for example, sits for long periods of time in a vibrating truck and then often helps to unload the truck, lifting and straining at the end of the day. This explains why truck driving ranks first in workers' compensation cases for low back pain. Fire fighters also have a high incidence of low back pain, which has been related to such high-risk activities as operating charged water hoses, climbing ladders, breaking windows, and lifting heavy objects.

In general, for all workers, occupational risk factors include heavy lifting, lifting with bending and twisting motions, pushing and pulling, slipping, tripping or falling, and long periods of sitting or driving, especially with vibrations. Individual risk factors may include obesity, smoking, posture, psychological stress and anxiety, physical activity level, and degree of muscular strength and joint flexibility.

Prevention of low back pain has typically involved several recommendations, including these:

- Exercise regularly to strengthen back and abdominal muscles.
- Lose weight, if necessary, to lessen strain on the back. Most studies have shown that obese people are at a greater risk for developing low back pain.
- Avoid smoking. Studies have consistently shown that smokers have a risk of low back pain 1.5 to 2.5 times that of nonsmokers. Smoking appears to increase degenerative changes of the spine.
- Lift by bending at the knees, rather than at the waist, using leg muscles to do most of the work.
- Receive objects from others or from platforms that are near to the body, and avoid twisting or bending at the waist while handling or transferring the load.
- Avoid sitting, standing, or working in any one position for too long.
- Maintain a correct posture. (Sit with shoulders back and feet flat on the floor or on a footstool or chair rung. Stand with head and chest high, neck straight, stomach and buttocks held in, and pelvis forward.)
- Use a comfortable, supportive seat while driving.
- Use a firm mattress, and sleep on your side with knees drawn up or on your back with a pillow under bent knees.
- Try to reduce emotional stress that causes muscle tension.
- Be thoroughly warmed up before engaging in vigorous exercise or sport.
- Undergo a gradual progression when attempting to improve strength or athletic ability.

Education is the most common back pain prevention strategy used in industry. Many different types of programs, including comprehensive "back school" programs, provide information on how the back works and on preferred lifting techniques, optimal posture, exercises to prevent back pain, and stress and pain management.

## Treatment

Treatment of low back pain has proven to be complex and frustrating. The optimal management of low back pain is still under debate. Many nonsurgical treatments are available, but few have been proven effective or clearly superior to others.

Nonsurgical treatments include physical therapy (with exercise), strict and extended bed rest, trigger-point injections, spinal manipulation, epidural steroid injections, conventional traction, corsets, and transcutaneous electrical stimulation. Many treatments have been added to the list of ineffective treatments, with little guidance as to which ones are clearly effective.

Even physicians are confused. Back pain is one of the most common symptoms that lead people to visit a physician; yet according to a national survey by Dr. Daniel Cherkin of the University of Washington in Seattle, physicians vary widely in their beliefs regarding treatment of low back pain. "There was poor correspondence between the treatments physicians believed are effective and those that have been found effective by well-designed studies," concluded Dr. Cherkin. For example, a significant proportion of the physicians advocated strict and extended bed rest and traction to treat low back pain. There is now strong evidence that these treatments are ineffective.

## EXERCISE-HEALTH CONNECTION

### Is there a way to predict if I'm at risk for developing low back pain?

Although the evidence is not conclusive, there is growing support among experts that low trunk muscle strength is one factor that increases the risk for low back pain.

Despite the numerous causes and risk factors that have been related to low back pain, most attention has been directed toward viewing low back pain as a by-product of deficient musculoskeletal fitness. Many researchers feel that the combination of a weak back and a back-straining occupation greatly increases the risk of low back pain.

In particular, emphasis has been placed on the relationship of low back pain to weak abdominal and back muscles, and poor flexibility of lower back and hamstring muscle groups. Low back pain has been described as a disease of the sedentary lifestyle, and most fitness-testing batteries from professional organizations (e.g., the YMCA) include some version of a sit-up to evaluate abdominal strength/endurance as well as the sit-and-reach test to evaluate low back and hamstring flexibility.

Theoretically, weak muscles that are easily fatigued cannot support the spine in proper alignment. When a person stands, weak abdominals and inflexible posterior thigh muscles allow the pelvis to tilt forward, causing a curvature in the lower back (called lordosis). This places increased stress on the spine and a greater load on other muscles, leading to their fatigue. The tight hamstring muscles and lower back muscles combined with the weak abdominals can lead to the low back pain syndrome, say some experts.

A study in Japan, for example, showed that subjects with a prior history of low back pain had weaker trunk muscle strength and a "generalized muscular weakness" when compared to those who had not experienced low back pain. A study of youth in Finland found that a low level of physical activity and decreased spinal and abdominal muscle strength characterized those who developed low back pain. Many other studies have reported that patients with low back pain have low trunk muscle strength, reducing support and stabilization of the spine.

The evidence is far from conclusive, however, that poor musculo-skeletal fitness predicts low back pain among the general population. For example, in one study of 119 nurses, performance on fitness and back-related isometric strength tests did not effectively predict low back pain during an 18-month period. A 10-year study of 654 people in Finland failed to demonstrate any relationship between muscle function and the development of low back pain. In both adolescents and adults, flexibility measurements have been reported to have a low predictive value for the condition.

Dr. Amnon Lahad of the University of Washington in Seattle reviewed the literature on prevention of low back pain and concluded that "exercise interventions may be mildly protective against back pain. . . . There is limited evidence that exercises to strengthen back or abdominal muscles and to improve overall fitness can decrease the incidence and duration of low back pain episodes."

There is some indication, however, that low levels of musculoskeletal fitness are predictive of recurrent low back pain. In other words, when an individual of any age has a low back problem and then as a reaction engages in very little exercise, the likelihood of further episodes is enhanced. This can set up a vicious cycle, leading to chronic back problems.

*I never scored very well on the fitness tests I took in school, including the strength and flexibility tests. Is it true that those predict future low back pain?*

No. Most fitness experts have been unable to determine that these common fitness tests predict future low back pain.

For years, the one-minute timed, bent-knee sit-up has been used for measurement of abdominal strength/endurance, while the sit-and-reach test has been touted as a measure of low-back and hamstring flexibility.

However, there is no evidence that people who score low on both tests are at increased risk of low back pain in the future. Dr. Andrew Jackson, working with researchers at the Cooper Institute for Aerobics Research in Dallas, Texas, studied the effect of low scores on the sit-up and sit-and-reach tests on future low back pain. Nearly 3,000 adults were followed for seven years; those who scored low on these tests were not at increased risk for the development of low back pain.

*Is it dangerous to exercise if I have a bad back?*

In most cases, no, but there are times when back pain may signal that there is serious injury to the nervous system and that immediate medical assistance is crucial.

Experts recommend that a physician be seen immediately if the back pain

- follows an impact injury or some sort of fall or accident,
- follows lifting a heavy object when the lifter is elderly,
- is accompanied by a foot that slaps during walking or by inability to raise up on the toes,

- is accompanied by a continuous tingling, numbness, or weakness in the legs or lower trunk,
- is accompanied by a fever or chills, or
- is accompanied by loss of bowel or bladder control.

If the exercise or movement hurts, stop doing it until medical advice is obtained. If there is moderate to severe pain, wait until the symptoms lessen before beginning an exercise program. Each exercise session should be preceded by a gradual warm-up. Warm up the body by walking or riding a stationary bike for 5 to 10 minutes at an easy pace. This will warm the muscles and increase blood flow, making it easier to stretch.

Experts also recommend that most people with low back pain engage in low-stress activities such as walking, biking, or swimming during the first two weeks after symptoms begin, even if the activities make the symptoms a little worse. The most important goal is to return to your normal activities as soon as it is safe. Bed rest usually isn't necessary and shouldn't last longer than two to four days. More than four days of rest can weaken muscles and delay recovery.

---

### Will exercise help my back get better?

Extended bed rest is usually not necessary or beneficial in treating low back pain. The role of exercise remains controversial, however, with most experts advocating that a return to normal, daily activities is superior to either bed rest or specific back exercises.

---

Physical therapy with exercise is recommended by physicians more than any other nonsurgical treatment for low back pain (both acute and chronic). And yet according to most experts, the role of exercise in treatment of low back pain remains controversial. A recent review, for example, reported that only one of four well-designed studies has found a positive effect of exercise therapy in patients with low back pain.

In one of the earliest studies, Kraus and Raab used musculoskeletal exercises to treat 3,000 adult patients with chronic and acute back pain; they reported "good" improvement in 65 percent and "fair" improvement in 26 percent of the patients, but poor improvement in only 9.2 percent. In this study, however, no control group was utilized to determine whether patients engaging in no exercise at all would have experienced similar improvement.

Some researchers advocate an intensive back muscle-strengthening exercise program to treat low back pain. Patients can't exercise strenuously at first, but after various pain control measures are initiated, patients gradually progress through an increasingly difficult series of resistance exercises to improve back muscle strength.

In one study of 105 patients in Denmark with low back pain, 30 sessions of intense back extensor exercises over a three-month period led to significant improvement relative to groups exercising less intensely. These researchers have urged that training must be intensive and long term before significant decreases in back pain are experienced. This approach, however, is not accepted by the majority of low back pain experts; it is also time consuming and costly, requiring trained staff and hospital resources.

A study of 186 civil workers who sought treatment for acute low back pain in Helsinki, Finland, has provided some of the best data yet available regarding the relative merits of bed rest, exercise, and ordinary activity in the treatment of acute back pain. The patients were randomized to one of three groups: bed rest (for two days), exercise (back extension and side-bending movements), and normal activity (continuation of normal day routines within the limits permitted by their back pain).

As shown in figure 9.2, after three weeks those patients who maintained normal activities were significantly better off than those who had either rested in bed or exercised. Their back pain was less intense and didn't last as long, and they had missed fewer days on the job and felt better able to work. Recovery was slowest for the bed rest patients. As

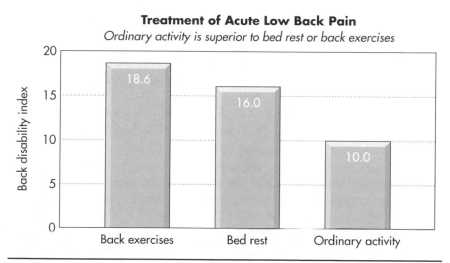

**Treatment of Acute Low Back Pain**

*Ordinary activity is superior to bed rest or back exercises*

FIGURE 9.2   Continuing ordinary activities leads to more rapid recovery of low back pain.

summarized by lead researcher Dr. Antti Malmivaara, "Our controlled study of workers with acute low back pain suggests that avoiding bed rest and maintaining ordinary activity as tolerated lead to the most rapid recovery. Widespread use of this approach in clinical practice would result in substantial monetary savings."

Most experts now feel that low back pain should be treated as a benign, self-limiting condition that usually requires little medical intervention. In a large study of close to 1,000 patients in Norway, Dr. Aage Indahl reported that "light and normal activity . . . and information and instruction designed to increase activity and reduce fear associated with the condition, had a significantly better effect on sickness leave than the ordinary medical practice in this community."

This conclusion is similar to that reached by a panel of 23 experts who reviewed nearly 4,000 studies on back pain, in a project sponsored by the federal Agency for Health Care Policy and Research. Among the agency's recommendations are these:

- Engage in low-stress activities such as walking, biking, or swimming during the first two weeks after symptoms begin, even if the activities make the symptoms a little worse. "The most important goal," the panel concludes, "is to return to your normal activities as soon as it is safe."

- Bed rest usually isn't necessary and shouldn't last longer than two to four days. More than four days of rest can weaken muscles and delay recovery.

- Nonprescription pain relievers such as aspirin and ibuprofen work as well as prescription painkillers and muscle relaxants and cause fewer side effects.

- Among treatments not recommended, due to lack of evidence that they work, are traction, acupuncture, massage, ultrasound, and transcutaneous electrical nerve stimulation.

- Diagnostic tests such as x-rays and computed tomography scans are rarely useful during the first month of symptoms, so they should be avoided during that time.

- Surgery helps only 1 in 100 people with acute low back problems. It should not be done during the first three months of symptoms unless a serious underlying condition such as a fracture or dislocation is suspected.

- Spinal manipulation by a chiropractor or other therapist can be helpful when symptoms begin, but patients should be reevaluated if they haven't improved after four weeks of treatment.

# REFERENCES

Battié, M.C., Bigos, S.J., Fisher, L.S., et al. (1990). The role of spinal flexibility in back pain complaints within industry. *Spine, 15,* 768-773.

Biering-Sorensen, F., Bendix, T., Jorgensen, K., Manniche, C., & Nielsen, H. (1994). Physical activity, fitness and back pain. In C. Bouchard, R.J. Shephard, & T. Stephens (Eds.), *Physical activity, fitness, and health: International proceedings and consensus statement* (pp. 737-348). Champaign, IL: Human Kinetics.

Cherkin, D.C., Deyo, R.A., Wheeler, K., & Ciol, M.A. (1995). Physician views about treating low back pain: The results of a national survey. *Spine, 20,* 1-10.

Dreisinger, T.E., & Nelson, B. (1996). Management of back pain in athletes. *Sports Medicine, 21,* 313-319.

Gundewall, B., Liljeqvist, M., & Hansson, T. (1993). Primary prevention of back symptoms and absence from work. A prospective randomized study among hospital employees. *Spine, 18,* 587-594.

Indahl, A., Velund, L., & Reikeraas, O. (1995). Good prognosis for low back pain when left untampered: A randomized clinical trial. *Spine, 20,* 473-477.

Kraus, H. (1965). *Backache, stress and tension: Their cause, prevention and treatment.* New York: Simon & Schuster.

Lahad, A., Malter, A.D., Berg, A.O., & Deyo, R.A. (1994). The effectiveness of four interventions for the prevention of low back pain. *Journal of the American Medical Association, 272,* 1286-1291.

Lee, J-H., Ooi, Y., & Nakamura, K. (1995). Measurement of muscle strength of the trunk and the lower extremities in subjects with history of low back pain. *Spine, 20,* 1994-1996.

Leino, P., Aro, S., & Hasan, J. (1987). Trunk muscle function and low back disorders: A ten-year follow-up study. *Journal of Chronic Diseases, 40,* 289-296.

Malmivaara, A., Häkkinen, U., Aro, T., et al. (1995). The treatment of acute low back pain—bed rest, exercises, or ordinary activity? *New England Journal of Medicine, 332,* 351-355.

Manniche, C., Asmussen, K., Lauritsen, B., et al. (1993). Intensive dynamic back exercises with or without hyperextension in chronic back pain after surgery for lumbar disc protrusion: A clinical trial. *Spine, 18,* 587-594.

Nuwayhid, I.A., Stewart, W., & Johnson, J.V. (1993). Work activities and the onset of first-time low back pain among New York city fire fighters. *American Journal of Epidemiology, 137,* 539-548.

Park, C., & Wagener, D. (1993). *Health conditions among the currently employed: United States, 1988* (National Center for Health Statistics, PHS 93-1412). Washington, DC: Government Printing Office.

Plowman, S.A. (1992). Physical activity, physical fitness, and low back pain. *Exercise and Sport Science Review, 20,* 221-242.

Ready, A.E., Boreskie, S.L., Law, S.A., & Russell, R. (1993). Fitness and lifestyle parameters fail to predict back injuries in nurses. *Canadian Journal of Applied Physiology, 18*, 80-90.

Salminen, J.J., Erkinalo, M., Laine, M., & Pentti, J. (1994). Low back pain in the young: A prospective three-year follow-up study of subjects with and without low back pain. *Spine, 19*, 2101-2108.

YMCA of the USA. (1994). *YMCA healthy back book.* Champaign, IL: Human Kinetics.

# Chapter 10

# ASTHMA

With the right medication plan, most asthma patients can participate fully in physical activities, including running and other exercise. Unlike other triggers, physical activity should not be avoided.

**Global Strategy for Asthma Management and Prevention,
National Institutes of Health/World Health Organization**

Tom Dolan stands six feet, six inches tall, weighs 180 pounds, and has just 3 percent body fat. His arms extend to hands that look like canoe paddles, and his size 14 feet could be classified as flippers. Swimming is natural to Tom except for one obstacle—exercise-induced asthma. If he didn't swim competitively, he might not even have known he had asthma, which in his case is induced solely by heavy exertion. But Dolan has learned to live with his asthma, and at the 1996 Olympic Games in Atlanta he won the gold medal in the 400-meter individual medley, an event in which he is also the world record holder.

Of the various triggers for asthma, physical activity is one of the most common. More than 80 percent of children and 60 percent of adults with asthma get exercise-induced asthma (EIA) during or after exercise.

## Pathology

Exercise-induced asthma was recognized as early as the second century A.D., when Aretaeus the Cappadocian noted, "If from running, gymnastic exercises, or any other work, the breathing becomes difficult, it is called Asthma." In 1698, Sir John Floyer, an English physician who himself had asthma, noted that the type of exercise (e.g., dancing vs. riding) affected whether or not asthma would be triggered. In the mid-1800s, the English physician Salter observed that EIA was aggravated by exposure to cold.

In 1946, medical researchers reported that the airways could constrict or tighten in response to fast breathing, and in 1963 it was shown that exercise could increase airway resistance in asthmatic children.

In the 1972 Olympic Games, EIA gained considerable attention when an American swimmer lost a gold medal due to the use of a banned drug to treat asthma. Recognition that EIA could be controlled with proper medication and education grew in the wake of reports of the success of U.S. Olympians. Of 597 U.S. athletes in the 1984 Olympic summer games in Los Angeles, 11 percent reported a history of EIA. These athletes still won 41 medals. In the 1988 Olympic games in Seoul, about 8 percent of U.S. athletes were confirmed asthmatics and won, proportionately, as many medals as did athletes without asthma.

Asthma (from Greek "to pant") is an inflammation of the lungs that causes airways to narrow, making it difficult to breathe. Inflammation makes the airways sensitive to allergens, chemical irritants, tobacco smoke, cold air, or exercise.

When a person is exposed to these stimuli, an asthma attack can occur, causing the muscles around the windpipes to tighten, making the opening smaller (see figure 10.1). The lining of the windpipe swells (becomes inflamed) and produces mucus. This leads to coughing, wheezing, chest tightness, and difficulty in breathing.

## Prevalence

Asthma symptoms come and go; they can last for a few moments or for days. Asthma attacks can be mild or severe, and sometimes fatal. Each year in America, more than 5,000 people die from asthma, with rates twice as high among blacks compared to whites.

Asthma is a major public health problem, affecting more than 100 million people worldwide and 5 percent of Americans (about 13 million). In the United States, about 1 child in every 15 has asthma. During the 1980s, for unknown reasons the asthma rates rose 49 percent, a problem now recognized in many other nations worldwide. According to experts of the Global Initiative for Asthma, "This may be linked to factors including housing with reduced ventilation, exposure to indoor allergens (such as domestic dust mites in bedding, carpets, and stuffed furnishings, and animals with fur, especially cats), tobacco smoke, viral infections, air pollution, and chemical irritants."

## Prevention

Asthma episodes can be prevented, but more studies are needed to determine whether or not development of the underlying inflammatory

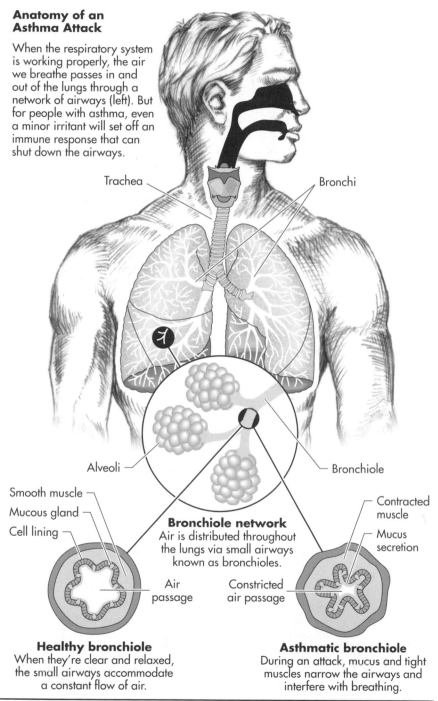

## Anatomy of an Asthma Attack

When the respiratory system is working properly, the air we breathe passes in and out of the lungs through a network of airways (left). But for people with asthma, even a minor irritant will set off an immune response that can shut down the airways.

Trachea

Bronchi

Alveoli

Bronchiole

Smooth muscle
Mucous gland
Cell lining

**Bronchiole network**
Air is distributed throughout the lungs via small airways known as bronchioles.

Air passage

Contracted muscle

Mucus secretion

Constricted air passage

**Healthy bronchiole**
When they're clear and relaxed, the small airways accommodate a constant flow of air.

**Asthmatic bronchiole**
During an attack, mucus and tight muscles narrow the airways and interfere with breathing.

FIGURE 10.1   The anatomy of an asthma attack.

disease can be averted. Controlling exposure to environmental allergens, irritants, and pollution may help prevent asthma. A California study of 3,000 nonsmokers between 1977 and 1992 showed that exposure to air pollution increased the risk of developing asthma. According to the American Lung Association, "This new research provides the strongest link yet between air pollution and asthma."

Asthma is no longer considered a condition involving isolated and periodic attacks. Rather, asthma is now understood to be a chronic inflammatory affliction of the airways. Inflammation makes the airways hypersensitive to a wide variety of irritants. Causes of the initial tendency toward inflammation in the airways are not yet known for certain, but one of the strongest risk factors is an inherited tendency to have allergic reactions.

Common allergens that are risk factors for developing asthma include house dust mites, animals with fur, cockroaches, pollens, and molds. Exposure to tobacco smoke, especially in infants, is a strong risk factor. Chemicals or air pollutants in the workplace can also lead to the development of asthma. Viral respiratory infections, small size at birth, and diet (e.g., certain foods such as shellfish, peanuts, eggs, and chocolate) may also contribute.

Many of these risk factors for developing asthma also aggravate it; these are known as triggers because they provoke asthma attacks. Other triggers include wood smoke from open fires or stoves, physical activity, extreme emotional expressions (laughing or crying hard), cold air, weather changes, certain food additives (e.g., metabisulphite, monosodium glutamate), and aspirin.

By avoiding triggers, a person with asthma lowers the risk of irritating the sensitive airways. The risk can be further reduced by taking medications that decrease airway inflammation.

Asthma can be intermittent, mild but persistent, moderate and persistent, or severe and persistent. Asthma differs between people and within a person over time. For example, asthma can be moderate in childhood and mild in adulthood, and for some people it is severe only during certain seasons.

Although asthma cannot be cured, it can be controlled by establishing a lifelong management plan with a physician. Patients can be educated to avoid triggers and use appropriate medications. Various quick-relief and long-term preventive medications should be considered. The quick-relief medications include short-acting bronchodilators (e.g., inhaled beta$_2$-agonists) that act quickly to relieve airway tightness and acute symptoms such as coughing, chest tightness, and wheezing. Long-term preventive medications (e.g., inhaled corticosteroids) help control the inflammation that causes attacks. Many asthma medications are delivered by metered dose inhalers, which are highly effective.

The best way to stop asthma attacks is prevention. Identifying and controlling triggers is essential for successful control of asthma. These are among the common triggers:

- **House dust mites:** These are often a major component of house dust; they feed on human skin sheddings. They are found in mattresses, blankets, rugs, soft toys, and stuffed furniture. Exposure to mite allergens in early childhood contributes strongly to the development of asthma. Hot laundering, airtight covers, removal of carpets, and avoidance of fabric-covered furniture are recommended.

- **Animal allergens from animals with fur:** Such animals include small rodents, cats, and dogs, and they can trigger asthma. Animals should be removed from the home.

- **Tobacco smoke:** Tobacco smoke is a trigger whether the patient smokes or breathes in the smoke from others.

- **Cockroach allergen:** This is a common trigger in some locations. Infested homes should be cleaned thoroughly and regularly.

- **Mold and other fungal spores and pollens:** These are particles from plants. Windows and doors should be closed, and it is recommended that persons with asthma stay indoors when pollen and mold counts are highest. Air conditioning can be helpful.

- **Smoke from wood-burning stoves and other indoor air pollutants:** Such smoke and pollutants produce irritating particles. Vent all furnaces and stoves to the outdoors, and keep rooms well ventilated.

- **Colds or viral respiratory infections:** Such infections can trigger asthma, especially in children. Patients with moderate to severe asthma should receive an influenza vaccination every year. At the first sign of a cold, asthma medications should be used to control symptoms.

- **Physical activity:** This a common trigger for most people with asthma.

## EXERCISE-HEALTH CONNECTION

Although the phenomenon is not entirely understood, most clinicians feel that EIA is triggered as the lining cells of the airway are cooled and dried during exercise. As air is taken into the lungs, it is warmed and humidified, resulting in a cooling and drying of the airway lining. Certain chemicals are then released by the lining cells, causing the airways to tighten. The cooling and drying are worsened by several factors, including exercising in cool and dry air, a switch from nasal to mouth breathing, and fast and deep breathing from intense exercise. If pollutants and pollen are in the air, the risk of EIA is increased.

---

### It seems logical to assume that exercise would trigger asthma attacks. Is that true?

Yes. Exercise-induced asthma is the temporary increase in airway resistance that develops in certain individuals after approximately five to eight minutes of strenuous physical exercise.

---

Symptoms of EIA do not generally occur during the exercise bout itself or during the first few minutes after exercise. Following exercise, EIA goes through at least three phases:

• **Early-phase response:** Within several minutes after a person stops exercise, the airways begin to tighten, leading to difficulty in breathing, wheezing, coughing, and chest tightness. The symptoms are most severe within 5 to 10 minutes after exercise. The EIA attack generally lasts 5 to 15 minutes.

In the laboratory, clinicians diagnose EIA if the ability to exhale a certain amount of air from the lungs quickly (within one second) falls by 15 percent or more after six to eight minutes of high-intensity exercise (90 percent of the maximal heart rate). (See figure 10.2.) Many people who have asthma now use peak-flow meters, which are small devices that measure how well air moves out of the airways. People with asthma should avoid exercising vigorously until the peak-flow reading returns to, or exceeds 80 percent of, the personal best peak-flow reading.

• **Spontaneous recovery:** Symptoms of EIA gradually diminish, usually within 45 to 60 minutes.

• **Refractory period:** If the individual exercises again within 30 to 90 minutes of the first bout, the airway tightening is markedly less, and fewer EIA symptoms are experienced.

Some individuals with EIA appear to experience a late asthmatic attack about three to six hours after the first one. This late response is still debated, and many factors other than exercise may be responsible.

Even though exercise may trigger asthma, the benefits that come from regular physical training are so important that most asthma experts urge that it be included as an important part of the management strategy of

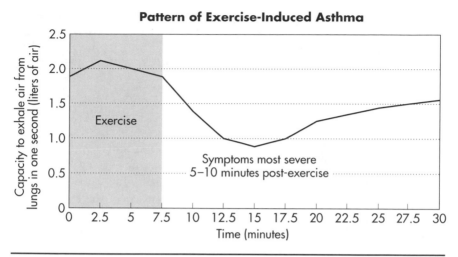

**Pattern of Exercise-Induced Asthma**

FIGURE 10.2   People with EIA experience wheezing, coughing, and difficulty breathing shortly after exercising.

asthmatic persons. "In the past, doctors discouraged people with asthma from exerting themselves to avoid triggering an attack. But the current thinking is that it is important for asthmatics to engage in regular exercise to condition and strengthen their lungs," says Dr. Stanley Szefler, director of clinical pharmacology at the National Jewish Center for Immunology and Respiratory Medicine in Denver.

---

### Can exercise-induced asthma be prevented or controlled?

With the right medication plan, most asthma patients can participate fully in physical activities, including running and other exercise. Unlike other triggers, physical activity should not be avoided. People with asthma who exercise regularly should monitor air flow with a peak-flow meter, avoid allergic triggers, use medication before exercise, and modify exercise habits and practices when necessary.

---

Regular exercise improves the overall physical fitness level of the individual with asthma, improves psychological mood state, decreases the risk for other chronic diseases, and improves heart and lung function. Also, several researchers have shown that as the person with asthma becomes physically fit, EIA attacks are less frequent.

Many famous athletes have coped with asthma, including Jackie Joyner-Kersee, Bill Koch, Greg Louganis, Dominique Wilkins, Jim Ryan, Tom Dolan, and Nancy Hogshead. Each learned how to follow his or her own personal asthma management plan, which included a mix of proper medications and control of asthma triggers.

Dr. Claude Lenfant, Director of the National Heart, Lung, and Blood Institute, has urged that students in particular be physically active. "Lifelong physical fitness is an important goal for all students," emphasizes Dr. Lenfant. "Yet students with asthma frequently restrict their physical activities. Much of this restriction is unnecessary—children with asthma can and should be physically active." The National Heart, Lung, and Blood Institute's National Asthma Education and Prevention Program encourages a partnership among students, families, physicians, and school personnel in managing and controlling asthma so that students can be active.

Individuals who follow their asthma management plans and keep their asthma under control can usually participate vigorously in the full range of sport and physical activities. Proper management of EIA includes

- monitoring air flow with a peak-flow meter,
- avoiding allergic triggers,
- using medication before exercise, and
- modifying exercise habits and practices.

A person's asthma symptoms can change a lot. They are often worse at night than during the day. They may be more intense in the winter or during "allergy seasons" when pollen counts are high. To help monitor airflow, the new National Heart, Lung, and Blood Institute guidelines include the recommendation that people with moderate to severe asthma use a peak-flow meter twice a day. Often decreases in airflow can provide an early warning of an asthma attack.

Drugs that relax the muscle spasm in the wall of the airways and help to open them (e.g., bronchodilators) are often the first line of treatment in preventing EIA. Doctors recommend using the medication (typically $beta_2$-agonist) from five minutes to an hour before exercise. $Beta_2$-agonist medications will control EIA in more than 80 percent of people with asthma and are helpful for several hours. However, because effectiveness does decrease with time, it is preferable to take the medication just before exercise. If breathing problems develop during exercise, a second dose may be needed.

Cromolyn sodium is often prescribed to treat athletes who have EIA. This drug, which is also an inhalant, prevents the lining of the airways from swelling in response to cold air or allergic triggers. Cromolyn sodium can be used up to 15 minutes before a person engages in physical activity. Corticosteroids should be used as preventive medicine, usually on an ongoing basis, to help control the underlying inflammation.

In addition to the use of proper medications, control of triggers, and use of peak-flow meters, several modifications to the exercise program have proven valuable:

- **Adequate warm-up and cool-down periods:** These help prevent or lessen episodes of EIA. The warm-up helps the individual with asthma take advantage of the refractory period in which episodes of EIA are reduced.

- **Type of exercise:** The form of exercise plays a critical role in determining the degree of EIA. Outdoor running is regarded as most conducive to EIA, followed by treadmill running, cycling, walking, and swimming. Swimming rarely leads to EIA because warm and humid air near the surface of the water prevents cooling and drying of the airways.

- **Length of exercise:** Long, intense, continuous exercise (e.g., running and cycling) causes more EIA than do repeated short bursts of exercise (generally less than five minutes each). Stop-and-go sports like tennis, volleyball, or football may lead to less EIA for some people with asthma.

- **Intensity of exercise:** High-intensity exercise (above 80 to 90 percent of the maximum heart rate) causes more EIA than does exercise at more moderate levels (e.g., walking).

- **Nasal breathing:** People with EIA should breathe slowly through the nose whenever possible. Nasal breathing warms and humidifies the air better than breathing through the mouth. Interestingly, research has shown that while breathing through the nose only, most people can reach an exercise intensity great enough to improve aerobic fitness.

- **Wearing a mask or scarf in cold weather:** This can increase the temperature and humidity of the inhaled air, reducing cooling and drying of the airway lining.

- **Monitoring the environment for potential allergens and irritants:** Examples include a recently mowed field, refinished gym floor, smoke in the air, or high pollen counts on a spring morning.

If an allergen or irritant is present, a temporary change in time of day or location should be considered because the presence of irritants can trigger more severe EIA attacks.

# REFERENCES

Donahue, J.G., Weiss, S.T., Livingston, J.M., Goetsch, M.A., Greineder, D.K., & Platt, R. (1997). Inhaled steroids and the risk of hospitalization for asthma. *Journal of the American Medical Association, 277*, 887-891.

Giesbrecht, G.G., & Younes, M. (1995). Exercise- and cold-induced asthma. *Canadian Journal of Applied Physiology, 20*, 300-314.

Hendrickson, C.D., Lynch, J.M., & Gleeson, K. (1993). Exercise induced asthma: A clinical perspective. *Lung, 172*, 1-14.

Mahler, D.A. (1993). Exercise-induced asthma. *Medicine and Science in Sports and Exercise, 25*, 554-561.

McKenzie, D.C. (1991). The asthmatic athlete: A brief review. *Clinical Journal of Sport Medicine, 1*, 110-114.

Papazian, R. (1994, January-February). Being a sport with exercise-induced asthma. *FDA Consumer*, 30-33.

Rupp, N.T. (1996). Diagnosis and management of exercise-induced asthma. *The Physician and Sportsmedicine, 24* (1), 77-87.

U.S. Department of Health and Human Services, PHS, NIH, NHLBI. (1991). *Guidelines for the diagnosis and management of asthma* (NIH Publication No. 91-3042). Bethesda, MD: National Heart, Lung, and Blood Institute.

U.S. Department of Health and Human Services, PHS, NIH, NHLBI. (1995). *Asthma and physical activity in the school* (NIH Publication No. 95-3651). Bethesda, MD: National Heart, Lung, and Blood Institute Information Center.

U.S. Department of Health and Human Services, PHS, NIH, NHLBI. (1995). *Asthma management and prevention, global initiative for asthma: A practical guide for public health officials and health care professionals* (NIH Publication No. 96-3659A). Bethesda, MD: National Heart, Lung, and Blood Institute.

Weiss, K.B., & Wagener, D.K. (1990). Changing patterns of asthma mortality: Identifying target populations at high risk. *Journal of the American Medical Association, 264*, 1683-1687.

# Chapter 11

# INFECTION AND THE IMMUNE SYSTEM

Research has shown that during moderate exercise, several positive changes occur in the immune system. Although the immune system returns to pre-exercise levels very quickly after the exercise session is over, each session represents a boost that appears to reduce the risk of infection over the long term.

Current Comment, American College of Sports Medicine

Sir William Osler, the famous Canadian medical doctor, once quipped, "There's only one way to treat the common cold—with contempt." Nearly 75 years have passed since that statement, but few physicians today can cough up any other opinion. Dr. George Jackson, one of America's leading cold researchers, admits that the common cold, "despite its frequency, has been something of an enigma to physicians and scientists."

## Prevalence

The U.S. Centers for Disease Control and Prevention has estimated that over 425 million colds and flus occur annually in the United States, resulting in $2.5 billion in lost school and work days and in medical costs. The average person has two or three respiratory infections each year, with young children suffering six to seven.

## Pathology

According to the Mayo Clinic, "A cold is an inflammation of the upper respiratory tract caused by a viral infection." The common cold is probably the most frequently occurring illness in humans worldwide. More than 200 different viruses cause colds, and rhinoviruses and coronaviruses are the culprits 25 to 60 percent of the time. Rhinoviruses often attack during the fall and spring seasons, while the coronavirus is common during the winter.

Although the mode of transmission is still a matter of controversy, growing evidence suggests that at least among adults, cold viruses are passed from person to person by being inhaled into the nose and air passageways (i.e., spread through the air). Severe colds transmit viruses more readily than mild ones because a greater amount of virus is passed into the air by coughing and sneezing. Thus to hinder the spread of cold viruses, coughs, sneezes, and "nose-blows" should be smothered with clean handkerchiefs or facial tissues.

Cold viruses are also spread by simple hand-to-hand contact with an infected person or with contaminated objects such as door knobs, telephones, or computer keyboards. Cold viruses can live for hours on hands and hard surfaces. When the hand is then brought to the nose or eyes, "self-inoculation" with the cold virus occurs. Thorough hand washing and the cleansing of counter spaces, handles, and knobs with Lysol or other disinfectants give protection against transmission. Also, keeping the hands away from the face is a good preventive measure. According to the Mayo Clinic, "Short of solitary confinement, the best you can do to prevent a cold is to wash your hands thoroughly and frequently with soap and warm water."

Damp, cold, or drafty weather does *not* increase the risk of getting a cold. According to most cold researchers, cold or bad weather simply brings people together indoors, which leads to more person-to-person contact.

## Treatment

Doctors will tell you that a cold lasts seven days without treatment, and one week with it. Most nonprescription medications, including antihistamines, decongestants, cough medicines, and analgesics, provide only temporary relief of symptoms. According to the Mayo Clinic, "Cold medications can make you more comfortable while you wait for your body to fight off the infection." To get rid of the cold, the body's immune system must make enough antibodies to destroy the viruses, a process that takes three or four days to get going. Antibiotics that fight bacteria have no value in the treatment of the uncomplicated common cold that is caused by a virus.

Even the old standby, inhaling steam, was found to have "no beneficial effect on the cold symptoms of our volunteers," says Dr. Gregory

Forstall of the Cleveland Clinic Foundation. Vitamin C, another common remedy, does not prevent colds, according to most researchers, but may slightly reduce the severity and duration of symptoms. Resting, drinking plenty of hot fluids, and seeking what comfort one can from over-the-counter cold remedies are still about all that can be done to treat most colds.

## Prevention

Whether or not one gets sick with a cold after a sufficient amount of the virus has entered the body depends on many factors that affect the immune system. Old age, cigarette smoking, mental stress, poor nutrient status, and lack of sleep have all been associated with impaired immune function and increased risk of infection.

Current knowledge suggests that good immune function can be maintained by eating a well-balanced diet, keeping life stresses to a minimum, avoiding chronic fatigue, and obtaining adequate sleep. Immune function is suppressed during periods of very low caloric intake and quick weight reduction, so weight loss should be gradual to maintain good immunity.

## EXERCISE-HEALTH CONNECTION

People who exercise report fewer colds than their sedentary peers. For example, a 1989 *Runner's World* survey revealed that 61 percent of 700 recreational runners reported fewer colds since beginning to run, whereas only 4 percent felt they had experienced more. In another survey of 170 experienced runners who had been training for 12 years, 90 percent reported that they definitely or mostly agreed with the statement that they "rarely get sick." A survey of 750 masters athletes (ranging in age from 40 to 81 years) showed that 76 percent perceived themselves as less vulnerable to viral illnesses than their sedentary peers.

---

*How does exercise affect my chances of getting a cold?*

Two randomized studies have provided important preliminary data in support of the viewpoint that moderate physical activity may reduce the number of days with sickness. A growing number of studies support the concept that after unusually heavy exertion or during overtraining, several components of immune function are negatively affected, increasing the risk for upper respiratory illness.

---

Very few studies have been carried out in the area of moderate exercise and colds, and more research is certainly needed to investigate this interesting question. Two randomized, controlled studies with young adult and elderly women have been conducted. In both studies, women in the exercise groups walked briskly for 35 to 45 minutes, five days a week, for 12 to 15 weeks during the winter and spring, while the control groups remained physically inactive. The results were in the same direction reported by fitness enthusiasts—walkers experienced about half the days with cold symptoms that the sedentary controls did (see figure 11.1).

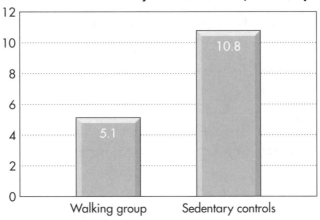

**Number of Sickness Days in 15 Weeks (Winter, Spring)**

FIGURE 11.1    Women walkers experienced half the sickness days of their sedentary peers.

Other research has shown that during moderate exercise, several positive changes occur in the immune system. Stress hormones, which can suppress immunity, are not elevated during moderate exercise. Although the immune system returns to pre-exercise levels very quickly after the exercise session is over, each session represents a boost that appears to reduce the risk of infection over the long term.

This has been likened to having a housekeeper come to the house every day for 35 to 45 minutes to tidy things up. By the end of the month, the house will be relatively clean and organized. In other words, every time an individual goes for a walk, the immune system receives a boost that should increase his or her chances of fighting off cold viruses over the long term.

Although public health recommendations must be considered tenta-tive, the data on the relationship between moderate exercise and lowered risk of sickness are consistent with guidelines urging the general public to engage in near-daily brisk walking.

Among elite athletes and their coaches, a common perception is that heavy exertion lowers resistance to colds. For example, Liz McColgan, one of the best female runners in Scotland, blamed overtraining, "which led to a cold and two subsequent illnesses," as the major reason for her poor performance in the 1992 World Cross Country Championships. Uta Pippig, winner of the 1994 Boston Marathon, caught a cold the week before the race after training 140 miles a week for 10 weeks at high altitude. Claimed Pippig, "When you are on such a high level you can so quickly fall off."

Alberto Salazar, once one of the best marathon runners in the world, reported that while training for the 1984 Olympic Marathon he caught 12 colds in 12 months. "My immune system was totally shot," he recalls. "I caught everything. I felt like I should have been living in a bubble." During the Winter and Summer Olympic Games, it has been regularly reported by clinicians that "upper respiratory infections abound" and that "the most irksome troubles with the athletes were infections."

To determine whether or not these anecdotal reports were true, researchers studied a group of 2,311 marathon runners who participated in the 1987 Los Angeles Marathon. During the week after the race, one out of seven runners came down sick, a rate that was nearly six times the rate for runners who trained for but did not run the marathon. During the two-month period before the race, runners training more than 60 miles a week doubled their odds for sickness compared to those training less than 20 miles a week. Researchers in South Africa have also confirmed that after marathon-type exertion, runners are at high risk for sickness.

The immune systems of marathon runners have been studied under laboratory conditions before and after running two to three hours. A steep drop in immune function occurs that lasts at least six to nine hours. Much of this immune suppression appears to be related to the elevation of stress hormones that are secreted in high quantity during and following heavy exertion. Several exercise immunologists believe this allows viruses to spread and gain a foothold.

Heavy training day in and day out has also been related to a chronic suppression of neutrophil function. This is a critical finding, because neutrophils are an important component of the immune system's "first-line defense."

Together, these studies on the relationship between exercise and infection have potential implications for public health, and for the athlete they may mean the difference between being able to compete or performing at a subpar level and missing the event altogether because of illness.

The relationship between exercise and infection may be modeled in the form of a J-curve. This model suggests that although the risk of infection may decrease below that of a sedentary individual when a person engages in moderate exercise training, risk may rise above average during periods of excessive amounts of high-intensity exercise (see figure 11.2).

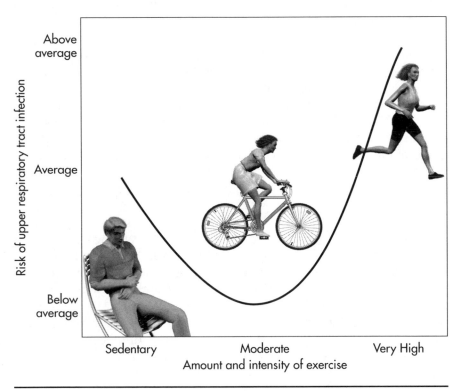

**FIGURE 11.2**   Moderate exercise may lower the risk of infection while heavy exertion may increase it.

## Is there anything I can do to reduce the risk of infection when I'm training hard?

Athletic endeavors are linked to many potential risks, including increased infection. Infection risk can be lessened in several ways by keeping other life stresses under control and reducing contact with cold and flu germs.

Athletes must train hard to prepare for competition. Although this increases the risk of infection if the training becomes too intensive, there are several practical recommendations the athlete can follow to minimize the impact of other stressors on the immune system:

- Keep other life stresses to a minimum. Mental stress in and of itself has been linked to an increased risk of upper respiratory tract infection.
- Eat a well-balanced diet to keep vitamin and mineral pools in the body at optimal levels. Although there is insufficient evidence to recommend nutrient supplements, ultramarathon runners may benefit by taking vitamin C supplements before ultramarathon races.
- Avoid overtraining and chronic fatigue.
- Obtain adequate sleep on a regular schedule. Sleep disruption has been linked to suppressed immunity.
- Avoid rapid weight loss (which has also been linked to negative immune changes).
- Avoid putting hands to the eyes and nose (which are primary routes for introducing viruses into the body). Before important race events, avoid sick people and large crowds when possible.
- For athletes competing during the winter months, flu shots are recommended.
- Use carbohydrate beverages before, during, and after marathon-type race events or unusually heavy training bouts. This may lower the impact of stress hormones on the immune system.

---

## Should I keep exercising if I am sick?

In general, if the symptoms are from the neck up, moderate exercise is probably acceptable and some researchers would argue even beneficial, while bed rest and a gradual progression to normal training are recommended when the illness is throughout the whole body (e.g., the flu). If in doubt as to the type of infectious illness, consult a physician.

---

Athletes and fitness enthusiasts are often uncertain whether they should exercise or rest during sickness. Human studies are lacking to provide definitive answers. Animal studies, however, generally support the finding that one or two periods of exhaustive exercise after the animal has been injected with certain types of viruses or bacteria lead to a more frequent appearance of infection and more severe symptoms.

With athletes, it is well established that the ability to compete is reduced during sickness. Also, several case histories have shown that sudden and unexplained downturns in athletic performance can sometimes be traced to a recent bout of sickness. In some athletes, exercising when sick can lead to a severely debilitating state known as post-viral fatigue syndrome. The symptoms can persist for several months and include weakness, inability to train hard, easy fatigability, frequent infections, and depression.

Concerning exercising when sick, most clinical authorities in the area of exercise immunology make these recommendations:

- If one has common cold symptoms (e.g., runny nose and sore throat without fever or general body aches and pains), intensive exercise training may be safely resumed a few days after the resolution of symptoms.

- Mild-to-moderate exercise (e.g., walking) when a person is sick with the common cold does not appear to be harmful. In two studies using nasal sprays of a rhinovirus leading to common cold symptoms, subjects were able to engage in exercise during the course of the illness without any negative effects on severity of symptoms or performance capability.

- With symptoms of fever, extreme tiredness, muscle aches, and swollen lymph glands, two to four weeks should probably be allowed before resumption of intensive training.

# THE ROLE OF EXERCISE IN HUMAN IMMUNODEFICIENCY VIRUS-INFECTED INDIVIDUALS

Although first recognized in 1981, acquired immune deficiency syndrome (AIDS) has become a major public health problem of this generation.

Within several weeks to several months after infection with the human immunodeficiency virus (HIV), many individuals develop a mononucleosis-like illness lasting a week or two. Most persons infected with HIV develop antibodies that can be measured within one to three months, although occasionally there may be a more prolonged interval.

Persons infected with HIV may be free of signs or symptoms for many months to years. Various symptoms progress to fully developed AIDS infection, which includes more than a dozen different infections and several cancers. Although the vast majority of HIV-infected persons develop AIDS within 15 or 20 years, with modern therapy the incubation period is expected to be considerably longer. Without therapy, about 80 to 90 percent of patients die within three to five years after diagnosis.

The primary target of this virus is the T-helper/inducer lymphocyte, an important cell of the immune system (see figure 11.3). The HIV attaches to a special marker on the T-helper cell called the CD4 antigen. The virus kills the T-helper cell as it divides. As a result, AIDS patients have a marked reduction in the number of T-helper or CD4 cells. When CD4 cell counts fall below 50 cells/mm$^3$, patients develop the most serious of the infections associated with AIDS. According to the Centers for Disease Control and Prevention, CD4 cell counts below 200 cells/mm$^3$ indicate the presence of AIDS.

---

## Can HIV be transmitted during sports?

No evidence exists for a risk of transmission of HIV when infected persons, without bleeding wounds or skin lesions, engage in sports.

---

Pertinent questions have been raised regarding HIV transmission during sports that require close physical contact. Most patients diagnosed with active AIDS are acutely and chronically ill and are not likely to participate in athletic endeavors. For each patient with clinically apparent AIDS, however, there are many more who are HIV infected and free of clinical symptoms who may be capable of normal participation in sports. Magic Johnson, formerly of the Los Angeles Lakers, is one of many examples.

Routine social or community contact with an HIV-infected person carries no risk of transmission; only sexual exposure and exposure to blood or tissues carry a risk. While the HIV has been found in saliva, tears, urine, and bronchial secretions, there is no evidence that the virus can be transmitted after contact with these secretions.

There are several situations, however, in which the transmission of HIV is of concern in athletic settings. In sports in which athletes can be cut, such as boxing or wrestling, or in other contact sports such as

**Symptoms and Effects of AIDS**

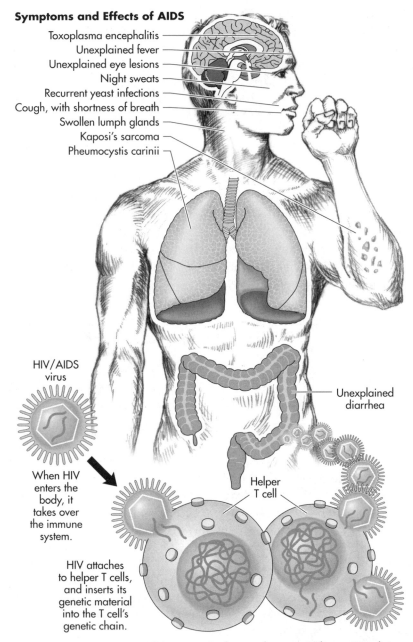

Toxoplasma encephalitis
Unexplained fever
Unexplained eye lesions
Night sweats
Recurrent yeast infections
Cough, with shortness of breath
Swollen lumph glands
Kaposi's sarcoma
Pheumocystis carinii

HIV/AIDS
virus

Unexplained
diarrhea

When HIV
enters the
body, it
takes over
the immune
system.

Helper
T cell

HIV attaches
to helper T cells,
and inserts its
genetic material
into the T cell's
genetic chain.

HIV can remain dormant for years. When activated, it
begins reproducing itself inside the T cell. These copies then
leave the T cell and enter the bloodstream, where they
attach to more T cells. The immune system is destroyed.

FIGURE 11.3   The anatomy of AIDS.

football, basketball, and baseball, risk of HIV transmission exists when the mucous membranes of a healthy athlete are exposed to the blood of an infected athlete. At present, the feeling is that testing all athletes prior to sport participation is impractical, unethical, and unrealistic. Therefore, the team physician and athletic trainer are urged to provide information about the transmission of HIV, recommended behaviors to reduce risks, and referral for care or diagnosis.

These concerns and concepts have been summarized in several professional reports:

• No evidence exists for a risk of transmission of HIV when infected persons, without bleeding wounds or skin lesions, engage in sports. Thus athletes infected with HIV should be allowed to participate in all competitive sports.

• There is no medical or public health justification for testing or screening for HIV infection prior to participation in sport activities. HIV testing should remain voluntary.

• There is a very low risk of HIV transmission during combative sports when an infected athlete with a bleeding wound or an oozing skin lesion comes in contact with another athlete who has a skin lesion or an exposed mucous membrane. Olympic sports with the greatest risk include boxing, tae kwon do, and wrestling, while basketball, field and ice hockey, judo, soccer, and team handball pose only moderate risk.

• It should be the responsibility of any athlete participating in a combative sport who has a wound or other skin lesion to report it immediately to a responsible official and seek medical attention. Athletes who know they are HIV infected should seek medical counseling about further participation in sports, especially in sports such as wrestling or boxing that involve a high theoretical risk of infection to other athletes.

• Each coach and athletic trainer should receive training in how to clean skin and athletic equipment surfaces exposed to blood or other body fluids.

• Gloves should be worn when contact with blood or other body fluids is anticipated, and skin surfaces should be washed and cleaned with soap and a diluted solution of household bleach (1:10 dilution) immediately if contaminated.

• Matches should be interrupted when an athlete has a wound where a large amount of exposed blood is present in order to allow the blood flow to be stopped and the area and athletes to be cleaned.

• Open wounds should be covered with dressings to prevent contamination.

- Athletes and officials in the high-risk sports should wear protective eyewear to reduce the possibility of bloody body fluids entering the eyes.

---

### Could exercise delay the development of AIDS in a person who is HIV positive?

No, but regular exercise is still recommended because it may improve life quality and psychological coping of HIV-infected individuals.

---

Very few studies have been published to provide an answer to this question. Surveys have generally found that long-surviving persons with AIDS exercise faithfully. However, many other factors besides exercise may explain their ability to live with AIDS.

Lawrence Rigsby (himself an AIDS patient) studied the effects of an exercise program (three one-hour sessions per week of strength-training and aerobic exercise) on 37 HIV-infected subjects who spanned the range of HIV disease from no symptoms to a diagnosis of AIDS (CD4 counts ranged from 9 to 804 cells/mm$^3$). Subjects were randomly assigned to either a 12-week exercise training or a counseling control group. Although exercise training had the expected effect in improving both strength and cardiorespiratory fitness in exercise subjects, no significant change in T-helper (CD4) cell counts was found.

During AIDS, patients often lose substantial amounts of body weight and muscle mass. Investigators have shown that weight training can help retard this "wasting syndrome" and improve life quality.

One conclusion that can be drawn from these studies is that appropriately supervised exercise training does not adversely affect HIV-infected individuals. Several potential benefits of both aerobic and strength training by HIV-infected individuals, especially when initiated early in the disease state, include improvement in psychological coping and the maintenance of health and physical function for a longer period. Improved quality of life is perhaps the chief benefit of regular exercise by HIV-infected patients, but there is no evidence that they should expect beneficial effects to their T-helper cells.

## REFERENCES

Mayo Clinic. The common cold. *Mayo Clinic Health Letter, 10,* 1-3.

Müns, G. (1993). Effect of long-distance running on polymorphonuclear neutrophil phagocytic function of the upper airways. *International Journal of Sports Medicine, 15,* 96-99.

Nieman, D.C. (1994). Exercise, upper respiratory tract infection, and the immune system. *Medicine and Science in Sports and Exercise, 26,* 128-139.

Nieman, D.C. (1996). The immune response to prolonged cardiorespiratory exercise. *American Journal of Sports Medicine, 24,* S98-S103.

Nieman, D.C., Henson, D.A., Gusewitch, G., Warren, B.J., Dotson, R.C., Buttterworth, D.E., and Nehlsen-Cannarella, S.L. (1993). Physical activity and immune function in elderly women. *Medicine and Science in Sports and Exercise, 25,* 823-831.

Nieman, D.C., Johanssen, L.M., Lee, J.W., Cermak, J., and Arabatzis, K. (1990). Infectious episodes in runners before and after the Los Angeles Marathon. *Journal of Sports Medicine and Physical Fitness, 30,* 316-328.

Nieman, D.C., Nehlsen-Cannarella, S.L., Markoff, P.A., Balk-Lamberton, A.J., Yang, H., Chritton, D.B.W., Lee, J.W., and Arabatzis, K. (1990). The effects of moderate exercise training on natural killer cells and acute upper respiratory tract infections. *International Journal of Sports Medicine, 11,* 467-473.

Pedersen, B.K., & Ullum, H. (1994). NK cell response to physical activity: Possible mechanisms of action. *Medicine and Science in Sports and Exercise, 26,* 140-146.

Peters, E.M., Goetzsche, J.M., Grobbelaar, B., and Noakes, T.B. (1993). Vitamin C supplementation reduces the incidence of postrace symptoms of upper-respiratory-tract infection in ultramarathon runners. *American Journal of Clinical Nutrition, 57,* 170-174.

Pyne, D.B. (1994). Regulation of neutrophil function during exercise. *Sports Medicine, 17,* 245-258.

Rigsby, L.W, Dishman, R.K., Jackson, A.W., Maclean, G.S., & Raven, P.B. (1992). Effects of exercise training on men seropositive for the human immunodeficiency virus-1. *Medicine and Science in Sports and Exercise, 24,* 6-12.

Shephard, R.J., & Shek, P.N. (1994). Infectious diseases in athletes: New interest for an old problem. *Journal of Sports Medicine and Physical Fitness, 34,* 11-21.

# Chapter 12

# CIGARETTE SMOKING

Smokers who get involved in aerobic exercise become
more aware of how smoking has decreased their ability to
process oxygen. In short, they find they become winded
more easily than their fellow exercisers. This helps create
a desire to quit smoking.

Dr. Kenneth H. Cooper

Pikes Peak looms 14,110 feet in the Colorado sky. Although the U.S.
Army explorer Zebulon Pike deemed this summit impossible to attain,
climbers now regularly take the narrow, precipitous 28-mile trail from
Manitou Springs to the peak and back. Each August more than 1,000
runners challenge the mountain during the Pikes Peak Marathon, one of
the oldest marathon race events in the United States. Only the fittest
runners who train year-round on the highest mountain ranges are able
to run the entire way to the top and back. Most end up mixing walking
with running as the thin air near the top leaves them gasping and light-
headed from lack of oxygen.

The Pikes Peak Marathon was first staged in 1956 by Dr. Arne
Suominen, an early critic of cigarette smoking. He was interested in
testing his theory, novel at that time, that cigarette smoking considerably diminished one's physical endurance. He challenged cigarette
smokers to race 10 nonsmokers to the top and back. Although three
smokers took up the challenge, none were able to finish the race as
Monte Wolford, a nonsmoking vegetarian, dominated the race from
start to finish. Despite repeated attempts, no smoker has ever won the
race, and according to most fitness experts, none ever will.

# SMOKING-RELATED DISEASES

The Surgeon General regards cigarette smoking as "the single most preventable cause of premature death in the United States." On January 11, 1964, the Surgeon General released the first report on smoking and health, concluding that "cigarette smoking is causally related to lung cancer." This historic report was widely covered by the media and created an immediate outcry from the tobacco industry that continues unabated to the present.

The Department of Health and Human Services has ranked tobacco as the leading underlying cause of death in the United States today followed by diet and inactivity, and then alcohol (see figure 12.1). Nearly one out of every five deaths is the result of cigarette smoking, with over 400,000 smokers dying each year from heart disease, cancer, and other diseases. An additional 10 million American smokers suffer from various debilitating diseases including bronchitis, emphysema, ulcers, and "hardening of the arteries." The decision not to smoke adds an average of 15 years of life in comparison to the shortened life expectancy of those electing to smoke.

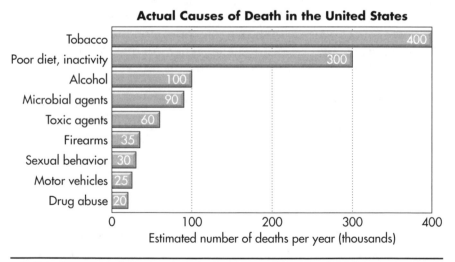

**Actual Causes of Death in the United States**

Estimated number of deaths per year (thousands)

- Tobacco: 400
- Poor diet, inactivity: 300
- Alcohol: 100
- Microbial agents: 90
- Toxic agents: 60
- Firearms: 35
- Sexual behavior: 30
- Motor vehicles: 25
- Drug abuse: 20

FIGURE 12.1   Use of tobacco ranks highest in actual causes of death in the U.S.

The major cause of death of smokers is coronary heart disease, with rates for heavy smokers about three times greater than in nonsmokers. At every level of serum cholesterol or blood pressure, smoking doubles or triples the death rate from coronary heart disease. Smokers with high blood cholesterol and blood pressure levels have coronary heart disease death rates that are about 20 times greater than for nonsmokers with low levels.

## Prevalence

The proportion of U.S. adults who smoke has fallen strongly since the 1960s, such that today only one in four still has the habit. However, the Year 2000 goal of 20 percent is unlikely to be met because little decrease in smoking prevalence has occurred since 1990. Cigarette smoking is still a major problem among blue-collar workers, those with little education, and various minority groups.

Cigarette smoking almost always begins in the adolescent years. It has been estimated that more than one million young persons start to smoke each year, adding about $10 billion during their lifetimes to the cost of health care in the United States. The prevalence of tobacco use among adolescents is increasing, with one of three high school students reporting current cigarette use.

In contrast, overall per capita consumption of cigarettes peaked during the 1960s around the time of the first Surgeon General's report and has since fallen strongly, especially during the 1980s. Social forces and legislation have had a strong impact. Public attitudes toward smoking have changed, much of the change due to the recent evidence that many adverse health effects are related to passive smoking (breathing someone else's cigarette smoke). The National Cancer Institute has concluded that "there is no longer any doubt that exposure to environmental tobacco smoke (ETS) is a cause of death and disease among nonsmokers."

Adults are quitting smoking cigarettes in huge numbers, with nearly half of all "ever smokers" now "former smokers." Most smokers report that they want to stop using cigarettes but have an extremely difficult time stopping, explaining why 46 million Americans are still current smokers. The Surgeon General has stated that cigarettes and other forms of tobacco are addicting in the same sense as are heroin, cocaine, and other drugs.

# SMOKING CESSATION

Smoking cessation methods fall into two major categories:

• **Self-help strategies**—quitting abruptly and completely, using manuals or nonprescription drugs. Approximately 90 percent of successful quitters have used a self-help strategy, most by quitting abruptly.

• **Assisted strategies**—use of smoking cessation clinics, hypnosis, acupuncture, or nicotine gum or patch with counseling. In 1992, a new product, the nicotine patch, was introduced, and it has been shown to produce six-month quit rates of 22 to 42 percent in comparison with 5 to 28 percent for placebo patches. Nicotine patches appear to reduce some, but not all, of the nicotine withdrawal symptoms. For example, while the patch reduces craving for cigarettes and negative moods, it does not appear to reduce hunger or weight gain. The nicotine patch should be used for six to eight weeks, and is most effective when appropriate support counseling is given.

According to the Surgeon General, there are many benefits to the smoker who quits:

• **Reduced overall death rates:** After 15 years off cigarettes, the risk of death from all causes for ex-smokers returns to nearly the level of persons who have never smoked.

• **Reduced heart disease risk:** After just one year off cigarettes, the excess risk of heart disease caused by smoking is reduced by half.

• **Reduced lung cancer risk:** The risk of lung cancer for ex-smokers drops to as much as one-half that of continuing smokers after 10 years. Risk of many other cancers is also lowered.

• **Improved life quality:** Ex-smokers have fewer days of illness and health complaints, better overall health status, and fewer lung problems. Ex-smokers can exercise more easily, feel better about themselves, and experience an increased sense of control.

## EXERCISE-HEALTH CONNECTION

Smoking and sports do not mix, and today it is quite rare to find an elite athlete who smokes. When Michael Jordan, who does not smoke, won his first National Basketball Association title, *Sports Illustrated* put him on the cover with a cigar in his mouth, prompting many readers to scold the magazine for portraying their icon in such a misleading fashion.

Surveys have shown that the prevalence of smoking is low among people who exercise. According to one study of 2,300 participants in the 1987 Los Angeles Marathon, only 3 percent were smokers. Among military personnel, researchers have shown that those exercising the most smoke the least.

The 1990 Youth Risk Behavior Survey showed that adolescents involved in vigorous physical activity and interscholastic sports had a much lower prevalence of smoking than those exercising little. Other studies have shown that youth who smoke exercise less than those who abstain, and that young smokers are prone to other high-risk behaviors such as drinking, drug use, carrying weapons, failure to wear seat belts, and engaging in physical fights.

---

### Does smoking affect how hard I can exercise?

Yes, most studies have shown that smoking decreases the ability to engage in vigorous and intense exercise.

---

The Surgeon General of the United States has conjectured that smokers are less likely than nonsmokers to make regular exercise a part of their lives, in part because exercise is more difficult. Many studies have established that smoking decreases the ability to perform vigorous exercise because of

- increased blood levels of carbon monoxide,
- decreased lung function, and
- decreased maximal oxygen consumption.

Carbon monoxide is present in cigarette smoke in large amounts and rapidly enters the blood, combining with the hemoglobin in the red blood cells. Normally the hemoglobin carries oxygen to the muscles and cells of the body. When carbon monoxide from cigarette smoke is present, about 5 percent of the hemoglobin is taken over for more than five hours. This decreases the delivery of oxygen to the muscles during vigorous exercise, making all effort seem more difficult than normal.

At rest, and to a smaller extent during exercise, nicotine from smoking cigarettes increases the heart rate and blood pressure, decreases heart blood output, and increases the oxygen demands of the heart muscle. During exercise, nicotine also increases levels of blood lactate, a substance that can make people feel fatigued or feel like quitting exercise when it rises high enough. In animal studies, nicotine has been found to decrease the ability to engage in long-endurance exercise like swimming or running.

The resistance to air flow after smoking is increased in the lung passageways, making it harder to deliver air and oxygen to the lungs during hard exercise. In some people, cigarette smoke can trigger asthma symptoms, making it nearly impossible to exercise until symptoms subside.

Scientists who have compared the fitness of smokers and nonsmokers report that smokers come out on the short end. Dr. Kenneth Cooper studied 1,000 young recruits in the Air Force, including smokers and nonsmokers. The ability to run as far as possible in 12 minutes (the famous "Cooper test") was directly related to the number of cigarettes smoked, with those smoking more than 30 cigarettes a day in the worst shape.

Dr. Terry Conway of the Naval Health Research Center in San Diego studied the physical fitness of more than 3,000 Navy personnel, 44 percent of whom were smokers. Dr. Conway found smoking "to be a detriment to physical readiness even among these relatively young military personnel." In Switzerland, nearly 7,000 military conscripts 19 years of age were studied, and performance in the 12-minute run was found to be inversely related to both the number of cigarettes smoked and the number of years with the habit (see figure 12.2).

A seven-year study of 1,400 Norwegians showed that physical fitness and lung function declined at a significantly faster rate in those who

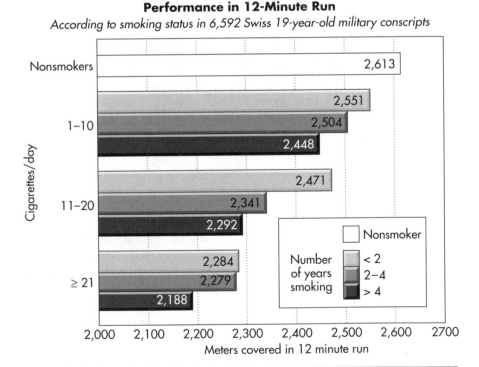

**Performance in 12-Minute Run**

*According to smoking status in 6,592 Swiss 19-year-old military conscripts*

FIGURE 12.2   The greatest decrement in 12-minute run performance is in heavy, long-term smokers.

smoked compared to nonsmokers. In other words, smokers are less fit to begin with because of their smoking, and then lose more fitness and lung function as time passes.

---

### Will a regular exercise program help me quit smoking?
Perhaps, but researchers have had a difficult time affirming this popular belief.

---

Dr. Cooper, now with the Cooper Institute for Aerobics Research in Dallas, Texas, has written that "smokers who get involved in aerobic exercise become more aware of how smoking has decreased their ability to process oxygen. In short, they find they become winded more easily than their fellow exercisers. This helps create a desire to quite smoking."

Proof of this assertion has been hard to come by, however. A cross-sectional study by the Centers for Disease Control and Prevention reported that 81 percent of male and 75 percent of female runners who had smoked cigarettes quit after beginning recreational running. Another study of 347 marathon runners, 38 percent of whom were former smokers, showed that about two-thirds of them claimed running had helped them to quit.

Other studies using better research designs, however, have produced conflicting results. Dr. Steven Blair of the Cooper Institute for Aerobics Research was unable to show that people increasing their physical fitness through regular exercise were more likely than nonexercisers to reduce smoking. A one-year, randomized, controlled, exercise training study of 160 women and 197 men by researchers at Stanford University failed to show any effect of exercise on smoking cessation.

However, in one study of more than 1,000 men and women who had participated in smoking cessation clinics at Kaiser Permanente medical centers, those who had increased their exercise after trying to quit were more likely to be nonsmokers one year later than those who had not. In another study of 2,086 smokers living in New England, those who were successful in quitting smoking were more likely than nonquitters to report efforts to increase exercise.

There's not yet conclusive evidence that exercise helps people stop smoking, but most smoking cessation programs include exercise as a vital component. "Exercise, such as walking, jogging, or bicycling," is included within the *Clinical Practice Guideline on Smoking Cessation* from the U.S. Department of Health and Human Services as a coping skill to handle stress and urges to smoke.

The Clinical Research Center at the Mayo Clinic includes exercise in its two-week comprehensive inpatient smoking cessation program for hard-core smokers. Also included are group therapy, stress management, daily lectures, supervised recreational activities, and nicotine patches. The one-year quit rate is 29 percent. Although it is not possible to separate out the effects of exercise, these clinicians along with many others view exercise as an integral part of smoking cessation efforts.

Nearly all smokers admit that their habit increases the risk of early death from cancer and heart disease, yet many are still unwilling to quit for fear of weight gain. The use of smoking as a weight-control strategy, risky though it may be, appears to be a powerful motivation for continued smoking for many people. In a nationwide survey in Australia, ex-smokers frequently listed weight gain as the number-one disadvantage of quitting.

---

## Will I gain weight if I stop smoking?

For most people who quit smoking, weight gain is modest and can be negated through prudent diet and exercise habits.

---

Cigarettes have long been associated with slenderness. As early as 1925, Lucky Strike launched its "Reach for a Lucky Instead of a Sweet" campaign, using testimonials from famous women such as Amelia Earhart and Jean Harlow. And the campaign continues, with advertisements today targeted to women with an emphasis on ultraslimness, sophistication, beauty, luxury, and popularity with men.

Unfortunately, there is an element of truth to these advertisements. Studies have established that the average smoker weighs about seven pounds less than a nonsmoker. People who start smoking lose weight, while those who quit gain, with women adding on an average of eight pounds and men six pounds. A 10-year study of 9,000 Americans by the Centers for Disease Control and Prevention confirmed that major weight gain (more than 28 pounds) can be expected in 10 percent of men and 13 percent of women who quit smoking. Two-thirds of all smokers who quit will gain weight, with the odds increasing for those who smoke more than 15 cigarettes per day. The researchers concluded that major weight gain is strongly related to smoking cessation, but that the average weight gain is rather small and unlikely to counter the health benefits of smoking cessation.

Not only do smokers tend to weigh less than nonsmokers, some studies even suggest they have less body fat despite eating the same

## What benefits can I expect from exercising while quitting smoking?

Exercise can help the former smoker improve physical fitness, lower risk of chronic disease, counter potential weight gain, and aid in coping with the symptoms of withdrawal.

amount while exercising less. It appears that smoking elevates the metabolic rate by 6 to 10 percent (about 200 calories) and that when people quit, the rate falls back down. And then if appetite and food intake are increased, as is commonly reported by those who quit, weight gain is inevitable. According to the Surgeon General, most studies show that food intake, especially of sweet foods, increases after quitting, resulting in 200 to 250 extra calories a day. This combined with the fall in metabolic rate translates to weight gain.

Although the issue has not been settled in careful research, most clinicians feel that regular exercise is particularly important for people quitting smoking. Each smoker should first seek physician approval to exercise to ensure that a safe exercise program can be started and maintained. There are four good reasons for encouraging exercise among former smokers:

• **Improvement in physical fitness:** Smokers typically have poor levels of fitness, and beginning a regular exercise program can improve heart and lung function and increase muscular strength and endurance.

• **Diminished risk of smoking-related diseases:** Regular exercise can decrease the levels of various risk factors and reduce the risk for heart disease and some cancers, helping to counter some of the negative disease consequences of smoking.

• **Countering weight gain:** Burning extra calories through exercise may help the quitter avoid the typical gain in weight. Walking about three miles a day burns the same amount of calories as smoking about a pack of cigarettes a day (but without the unpleasant and negative effects on health). So if a former smoker starts a daily walking program while seeking to avoid foods rich in fats and sugars, there is every reason to believe that weight gain can be avoided. Although two of three smokers who quit gain weight, one of three does not. An exercise program can improve the odds of joining the ranks of the no-gainers.

Although more research is needed, data from the Nurses Health Study at Harvard University support the notion that weight gain after smoking cessation can be minimized by even a modest amount of exercise.

- **Coping with stress:** Many individuals use smoking as a method of coping with stress and find the habit to be relaxing. Within two hours after quitting, typical feelings of nicotine withdrawal include irritability, frustration, anger, difficulty in concentrating, restlessness, depression, impatience, disrupted sleep, and impaired ability to work. These feelings peak within the first 24 hours and then gradually decline, usually subsiding within one month. The smoker who quits is faced with two psychological problems—the feelings of withdrawal from the nicotine in cigarettes and a loss of a useful method to cope with stress.

Regular exercise is an excellent substitute for smoking in improving psychological mood state and alleviating anxiety and depression, as well as in helping the quitter cope with some of the immediate negative mood states. Dr. Ken Cooper reported, "I have received hundreds of letters from cigarette smokers telling me how they could never break the habit until they started exercising."

For smokers who can't quit or refuse to quit, exercise is still encouraged to reduce risk of heart disease and early death. Exciting data from the Cooper Institute for Aerobics Research have shown that smokers who maintain a high level of physical fitness have lower death rates from all causes than do low-fitness nonsmokers. The lowest death rates, however, are found among men and women who avoid smoking while maintaining moderate to high physical fitness levels.

# REFERENCES

Blair, S.N., Goodyear, N.N., Wynne, K.L., & Saunders, R.P. (1984). Comparison of dietary and smoking habit changes in physical fitness improvers and nonimprovers. *Preventive Medicine, 13,* 411-420.

Blair, S.N., Kampert, J.B., Kohl, H.W., et al. (1996). Influences of cardiorespiratory fitness and other precursors on cardiovascular disease and all-cause mortality in men and women. *Journal of the American Medical Association, 276,* 205-210.

Brown, D.R., Croft, J.B., Anda, R.F., Barrett, D.H., & Escobedo, L.G. (1996). Evaluation of smoking on the physical activity and depressive symptoms relationship. *Medicine and Science in Sports and Exercise, 28,* 233-240.

Conway, T.L., & Cronan, T.A. (1992). Smoking, exercise, and physical fitness. *Preventive Medicine, 21,* 723-734.

Cooper, K.H. (1970). *The new aerobics.* New York: Bantam Books.

Cooper, K.H., Gey, G.O., & Bottenberg, R.A. (1968). Effects of cigarette smoking on endurance performance. *Journal of the American Medical Association, 203,* 123-126.

Derby, C.A., Lasater, T.M., Vass, K., Gonzalez, S., & Carleton, R.A. (1994). Characteristics of smokers who attempt to quit and of those who recently succeeded. *American Journal of Preventive Medicine, 10*, 327-334.

Erikssen, S.L., & Thaulow, E. (1995). Smoking habits and long-term decline in physical fitness and lung function in men. *British Medical Journal, 311*, 715-718.

Escobedo, L.G., Marcus, S.E., Holtzman, D., & Giovino, G.A. (1993). Sports participation, age at smoking initiation, and the risk of smoking among US high school students. *Journal of the American Medical Association, 269*, 1391-1395.

Kawachi, I., Troisi, R.J., Rotnitzky, A.G., Coakley, E.H., & Colditz, G.A. (1996). Can physical activity minimize weight gain in women after smoking cessation? *American Journal of Public Health, 86*, 999-1004.

Marti, B., Abelin, T., Minder, C.E., & Vader, J.P. (1988). Smoking, alcohol consumption, and endurance capacity: An analysis of 6,500 19-year-old conscripts and 4,100 joggers. *Preventive Medicine, 17*, 79-92.

McGinnis, J.M., & Foege, W.H. (1993). Actual causes of death in the United States. *Journal of the American Medical Association, 270*, 2207-2212.

Symons, J.D., & Stebbins, C.L. (1996). Hemodynamic and regional blood flow responses to nicotine at rest and during exercise. *Medicine and Science in Sports and Exercise, 28*, 457-467.

U.S. Department of Health and Human Services. (1990). *The health benefits of smoking cessation* (DHHS, PHS, Office on Smoking and Health, DHHS Publication No. (CDC) 90-8416). Washington, DC: Superintendent of Documents.

U.S. Department of Health and Human Services. (1994). Cigarette smoking among adults—United States, 1993. *Morbidity and Mortality Weekly Report, 43*, 925-930.

U.S. Department of Health and Human Services. (1996). Tobacco use and usual source of cigarettes among high school students—United States, 1995. *Morbidity and Mortality Weekly Report, 45*, 413-418.

Williamson, D.F., Madans, J., Anda, R.F., et al. (1991). Smoking cessation and severity of weight gain in a national cohort. *New England Journal of Medicine, 324*, 739-745.

Williard, J.C., & Schoenborn, C.A. (1995). Relationship between cigarette smoking and other unhealthy behaviors among our nation's youth: United States, 1992. *Advance Data from Vital and Health Statistics*, No. 263. Hyattsville, MD: National Center for Health Statistics.

# Chapter 13

# BLOOD CHOLESTEROL

Given that cigarette smoking appears to be declining and will perhaps become a rather unusual habit by the turn of the century, diet change, exercise, and their offspring, a lifelong healthy weight, will be the major hygienic weapons available to fight chronic disease and its depredations among our older population in the 21st century.

Dr. Peter D. Wood, Stanford University

Edith Brown was a subject in one of my studies who was randomized to the "walking only" group. Other subjects were appointed to the "diet only" (1,200 calories per day of healthy food), "diet and walking," and control groups (neither diet nor walking). Subjects in the walking groups walked 45 minutes, five days per week, at a brisk pace, for 12 weeks. Edith started the study with a blood cholesterol of 210 mg/dl and finished the study with a level of 212 mg/dl, and she was quite disappointed, not to mention surprised. Other members of the walking group had the same outcome, while those on the diet (with or without walking) experienced a strong decrease of 30 mg/dl (in concert with their loss of 20 pounds of body weight). In other words, 12 weeks of hard walking did not cause the blood cholesterol to drop, while weight loss did. Is it a myth that exercise lowers blood cholesterol? More on this later in the chapter.

## CHOLESTEROL FACTS

As reviewed in chapter 3, high blood cholesterol is a serious problem: It is a major risk factor for heart disease, the number-one killer of both men and women in the United States.

The body makes its own cholesterol and also absorbs cholesterol from certain kinds of foods, specifically all animal products (i.e., meats, dairy products, and eggs). Cholesterol is essential for the formation of bile acids (used in fat digestion) and some hormones, and is a component of cell membranes as well as brain and nerve tissues.

Thus some cholesterol is necessary to keep the body functioning normally. However, when blood cholesterol levels are too high, some of the excess is deposited in the artery walls, increasing the risk of heart disease. And in contrast, according to many studies, when blood cholesterol levels are lowered through lifestyle changes and medication, coronary heart disease decreases. In fact, for every 1 percent reduction in blood cholesterol, the occurrence of coronary heart disease is reduced 2 or 3 percent.

## Prevalence

Experts urge that everyone know his or her cholesterol level and have it checked at least once every five years (or every year if heart disease risk is high). Americans are more "cholesterol conscious" than ever before. A poll by the National Heart, Lung, and Blood Institute showed that 75 percent of Americans have had their cholesterol checked and that about half can recall their own cholesterol level. Blood cholesterol levels fall into one of three categories:

- Desirable:  less than 200 mg/dl
- Borderline high:  200-239 mg/dl
- High:  240 mg/dl and above

Despite an impressive drop from the 1960s, 20 percent of Americans still have high blood cholesterol levels, and 31 percent have borderline-high levels. The American average is 205 mg/dl, and if present trends continue, the Healthy People Year 2000 goal of 200 mg/dl will probably be achieved. Some populations around the world with very low risk of heart disease have blood cholesterol levels below 160 mg/dl, a zone now regarded by some experts as "optimal." In the Framingham Heart Study, for example, a study initiated during the 1950s, heart disease has been extremely rare among those with blood cholesterol levels within the optimal zone.

# "GOOD" AND "BAD" CHOLESTEROL

Cholesterol and other fats such as triglycerides are transported through the blood by carriers called lipoproteins. Two specific types of cholesterol carriers are called low-density lipoproteins (LDL) and high-density lipoproteins (HDL). (See figure 13.1.) High levels of LDL-cholesterol, sometimes called "bad" cholesterol, cause the cholesterol to build

## Functions of Lipoproteins

LDL and HDL have opposing functions. HDL takes cholesterol to the liver, where it is changed to bile and eventually excreted in the stool. This is the body's major method of reducing its cholesterol stores.

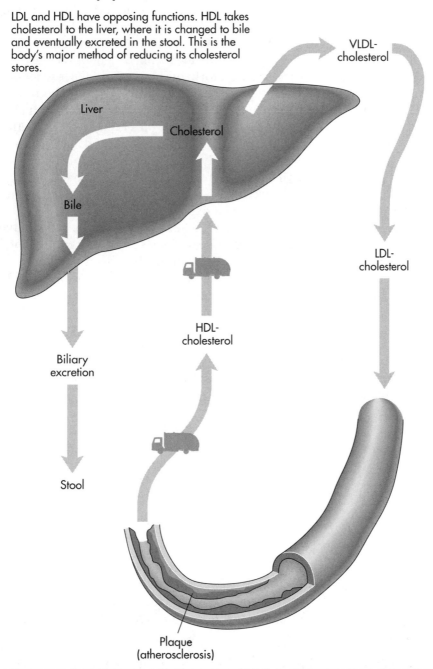

**FIGURE 13.1**   HDL acts as waste haulers, carrying cholesterol to the liver for processing. From *Fitness & Sports Medicine: A Health Related Approach* by David C. Nieman. Copyright © 1995 by Mayfield Publishing Company. Adapted by permission of the publisher.

up in the walls of the arteries, increasing heart disease risk. The level of LDL-cholesterol is classified as desirable if it is less than 130 mg/dl, borderline-high risk if 130-159 mg/dl, and high risk if 160 mg/dl and above. An optimal LDL-cholesterol level is 100 mg/dl or less.

In contrast, HDL-cholesterol, sometimes called "good" cholesterol, helps the body get rid of the cholesterol in the blood. The HDL carrier acts as a type of shuttle as it takes up cholesterol from the blood and body cells and transfers it to the liver, where it is used to form bile acids. Eventually, the bile acids pass out of the body in the stool, providing the body with a major route for excretion of cholesterol. For this reason HDLs have been called the "garbage trucks" of the body, collecting cholesterol and dumping it into the liver. Thus if levels of HDL-cholesterol are high (i.e., 60 mg/dl or above), the risk of heart disease is decreased. An HDL-cholesterol level of less than 35 mg/dl is considered low or undesirable.

Because of the importance of HDL-cholesterol, various ratios have been used to improve prediction of heart disease risk. The ratio of total cholesterol to HDL-cholesterol (TC/HDL-C) has been shown to be extremely useful in estimating heart disease risk, according to Dr. Steven Grover of the Montreal General Hospital in Canada. A ratio below 3.0 is considered optimal, while 5.0 and above is considered high risk. For every unit the ratio falls (e.g., 5.0 to 4.0), risk of coronary heart disease drops 50 percent. The average American adult male has a 4.6 ratio; the average female, 4.0. Elderly people, persons who are obese, and smokers have high ratios, while females, African Americans, and physically active people have lower ratios.

## Lifestyle Treatment

To have a favorable TC/HDL-C, the total cholesterol and LDL-C must be lowered and the HDL-C elevated through dietary and lifestyle factors. In order of importance, these are the factors that increase HDL-cholesterol:

- Aerobic exercise, at least 80 to 90 minutes per week
- Weight reduction and leanness
- Smoking cessation
- Moderate alcohol consumption

The most important factors for lowering LDL-cholesterol and total cholesterol are these:

- Reduction of dietary saturated fat intake (found mainly in meats, dairy products, and some tropical oils), with a greater emphasis on most plant oils and fish

- Reduction in body weight
- Reduction in dietary cholesterol intake (found in foods of animal origin)
- Increase in carbohydrates and dietary fiber (especially fruits and vegetables, beans, and oat products)

The status of blood triglyceride (i.e., fat) levels as a risk factor for heart disease is less clear. Most experts now feel that when borderline-high (200-399 mg/dl) or high (400 mg/dl and above) triglyceride levels are combined with low HDL-cholesterol levels, diabetes, obesity, and high blood pressure, the risk of heart disease is increased. Optimal triglyceride values are less than 110 mg/dl, with endurance athletes often having levels that fall below 80 mg/dl. Triglycerides can be lowered by losing weight, exercising aerobically, and reducing alcohol intake.

## EXERCISE-HEALTH CONNECTION

In the 1970s, several published studies showed that low levels of HDL-cholesterol were related to coronary heart disease. About the same time, the first reports that exercise may be related to improved HDL-cholesterol levels were published.

In an early study at Stanford University of male and female long-distance runners and sedentary controls (now considered a classic because of its far-reaching effects), HDL-cholesterol was found to be substantially higher in the runners. Total blood cholesterol, LDL-cholesterol, and triglycerides were reported to be much lower among the runners. But the researchers were unsure in this cross-sectional study (a research format that most experts regard as only a beginning point in the search for scientific truth) whether the group disparities in blood fats and lipoproteins were due to contrasts in exercise habits and/or differences in diet, body fat, and genetic background.

In two more recent and larger studies of male and female runners, a dose-response relationship between miles run per week and HDL-cholesterol was reported (see figure 13.2, a and b). In both of these studies, runners training the most had the highest HDL-cholesterol, and no evidence of a "plateau" or ceiling effect was seen. In other words, moderate amounts of running were better than little or none, while even more running was related to even higher HDL-cholesterol levels.

For the men but not the women runners, LDL-cholesterol and triglyceride levels dropped strongly with increase in running distance. However, once again, whether the improved blood lipoprotein profile among the more serious runners was due to genetics, or to a superior diet and body composition, could not be fully determined.

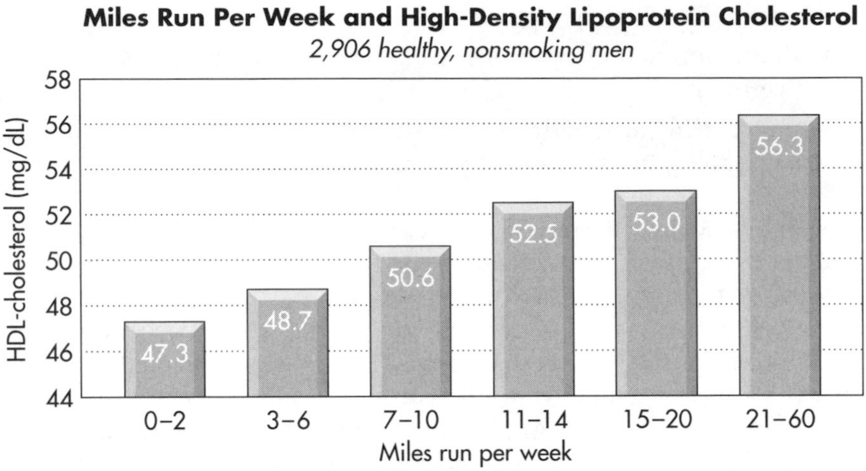

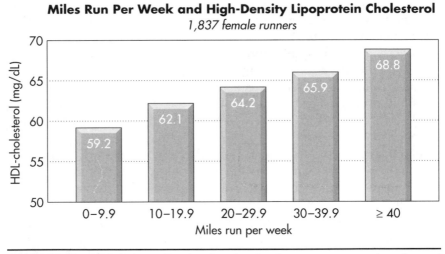

**FIGURE 13.2a**   Data indicate a dose-response relationship between miles run/week and HDL-cholesterol.

**FIGURE 13.2b**   HDL-cholesterol levels in females also show an increase as the miles run/week climb.

As emphasized in the first section of this chapter, weight loss, in and of itself, has a powerful effect on blood fats and lipoproteins. With weight loss the total cholesterol, LDL-cholesterol, and triglycerides decrease strongly, while HDL-cholesterol increases (but only when weight loss has been maintained and stabilized).

*Does exercise specifically improve cholesterol levels, or do cholesterol levels improve as an indirect result of the weight loss and dietary changes that usually accompany an exercise program?*

When separated from the effects of changes in body weight and diet, exercise training—especially when conducted frequently and intensively—has been shown to decrease blood triglyceride levels and increase HDL-cholesterol level, while having little or no independent effect on blood cholesterol and LDL-cholesterol.

Some researchers have estimated that the total cholesterol drops about 1 mg/dl for every pound lost (decreases are greatest for those with the highest blood cholesterol levels). In other words, if a woman changes her weight from 180 to 160 pounds, her blood cholesterol could be expected, on average, to decrease 20 mg/dl (e.g., from 205 to 185 mg/dl).

Dr. Leslie Katzel of the Baltimore Veterans Administration Medical Center conducted a nine-month study of 170 obese, middle-aged and older men who were appointed to weight loss, exercise training, or control groups. Subjects in the weight loss group lost on average 21 pounds, while the exercise group lost little weight but improved aerobic fitness by 17 percent after training intensively 45 minutes per session, three times a week. When looking across the entire blood lipid and lipoprotein profile, and considering other coronary artery disease (CAD) risk factors, Dr. Katzel concluded that "weight loss is the preferred treatment to improve CAD risk factor profiles in healthy, overweight, sedentary, middle-aged, and older men."

Improvements in dietary habits also have a favorable effect on blood lipids and lipoproteins. Going from the typical American diet to the one recommended by the American Heart Association can decrease the total cholesterol by 5 to 15 percent (depending on the initial level). Going to more extreme diets, like the 21-day Pritikin Program diet (<10 percent total fat), can have very strong effects on the total and LDL-cholesterol (20 to 25 percent decreases) and triglycerides (20 to 40 percent decreases). The Pritikin Program diet actually reduces HDL-cholesterol 10 to 20 percent, but the TC/HDL-C is not negatively affected. Researchers at the Pritikin Institute have reported that most of the improvements in blood lipids happen quickly, within the first two weeks, upon adoption of their low-fat, high-carbohydrate, high-fiber diet.

An even greater decrease in blood cholesterol level was reported by Dr. Roy Walford, chief medical officer of the Biosphere experiment near

Tucson, Arizona. Among eight subjects sealed inside this 3.15-acre space for six months, body weight fell 26 pounds in the men and 15 pounds in the women; during this time they ate a spare, vegetarian diet. Total cholesterol fell 36 percent (from 191 to 123 mg/dl). As with the Pritikin program, most of the improvements in blood lipids were experienced within the initial weeks.

Although most people will not go to these extremes, these studies do show that weight loss and dietary changes can have dramatic effects on the blood lipids and lipoproteins. Often when people begin exercise programs, improvements in dietary habits and body composition occur. Sorting out just which factor is responsible for the favorable changes in the various blood lipoproteins has challenged the best of researchers.

After the early cross-sectional studies on runners, additional studies at Stanford University, using randomized, controlled designs, have carefully demonstrated that changes in blood cholesterol and fats with exercise training are very much affected by parallel changes in body weight and diet. A growing consensus among investigators is that when changes in body weight and dietary habits are controlled for, exercise training alone can be expected to increase HDL-cholesterol and decrease triglyceride levels, with little or no effect on LDL-cholesterol.

How much exercise is necessary to produce this effect? Most experts in this area of research agree that an exercise program equal to a moderate jog or brisk walk for at least 30 minutes per session, three to five times per week, is necessary before improvements in HDL-cholesterol can be measured. In terms of energy expenditure, about 1,000 calories per week of moderate- to hard-intensity, aerobic-type exercise is required to produce favorable changes in blood fats and lipoproteins.

At this basic, minimum exercise level, changes in HDL-cholesterol and triglyceride levels are sometimes small and variable, depending on the individual. Exercise programs with high duration (e.g., 45 minutes or longer), intensity, and frequency (i.e., near daily) produce the strongest effects on HDL-cholesterol and triglycerides. Total cholesterol and LDL-cholesterol, however, appear to be little affected by exercise training, even when it is intensive, unless body weight is decreased or dietary saturated fats are lowered at the same time.

Figure 13.3 shows the results of one excellent study, conducted by Dr. Robert Schwartz of Harborview Medical Center in Seattle, in which changes in body weight and diet in both young and old men were minimized and controlled. After six months of training five days a week, 45 minutes per session, at a high intensity, aerobic fitness in the young and older subjects improved 18 and 22 percent, respectively. As shown in the figure, no significant changes in LDL-cholesterol were found

**Exercise & Lipoproteins in Young and Older Men Without Change in Weight/Diet**
*6 months exercise, 5 days/week, 45 minutes/session, high intensity*

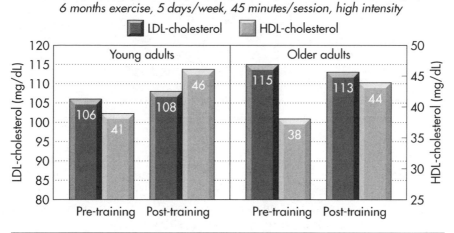

FIGURE 13.3  Both young and older men experience an improvement in HDL-C but not LDL-C with exercise when diet and weight loss are kept constant.

(because diet and body weight were kept near pre-study levels), while HDL-cholesterol improved 14 to 15 percent. Triglycerides were low in the young subjects before they started the study, so exercise training had no further effect. For the older subjects, triglycerides fell strongly.

---

### *Does exercise affect the cholesterol levels of men and women in the same way?*

Most studies have shown that women, who have higher HDL-cholesterol levels than men, require a greater volume of exercise to increase levels further.

---

Notice from figure 13.2 that female runners have higher levels of HDL-cholesterol than their sedentary peers despite the fact that women have higher levels than men to begin with. Also notice from figure 13.2, though, that men achieve gains in HDL-cholesterol at lower running distances than do women.

Many studies testing the effect of moderate amounts of walking on HDL-cholesterol in women have failed to show significant changes. However, when researchers increase the overall exercise volume and intensity, HDL-cholesterol does improve. In other words, women require greater volumes of exercise than men to improve their HDL-cholesterol because of the women's initially higher levels.

---

### How long do the benefits of exercise on cholesterol levels last?

Improvement in blood HDL-cholesterol levels are based on the day-to-day elevation that occurs after each exercise bout. After each exercise session, HDL-cholesterol rises and triglycerides fall; the degree of change depends on exercise duration and intensity and lasts for at least 24 to 48 hours.

---

Although there is increasing evidence that regular aerobic exercise increases HDL-cholesterol and lowers blood triglyceride levels, the exact mechanism explaining these positive changes is still being determined. At present, most researchers have concentrated their efforts on the interplay of important enzymes that regulate the breakdown and formation of HDL-cholesterol and triglycerides.

Regular exercise alters the activity of the regulatory enzymes in a favorable manner. The end result is that aerobically fit compared to unfit individuals appear to clear triglycerides from the blood more quickly, produce more HDL-cholesterol, and keep HDL in circulation longer.

Many studies have shown that single bouts of aerobic exercise, especially when prolonged and intense, result in immediate and significant increases in HDL-cholesterol. This acute increase in HDL-cholesterol has been linked to the breakdown of triglycerides during exercise. Certain enzymes (especially lipoprotein lipase in the walls of the capillaries) break down the triglycerides during exercise, allowing the muscles to take in fat for fuel and energy production.

As the exercise program is maintained on a regular basis, the acute changes in HDL-cholesterol and triglycerides, which persist for at least 24 to 48 hours, result in a "chronic" improvement. In other words, the favorable lipid profiles of trained individuals may actually be related to short-term changes that occur during or immediately after a single bout of exercise, which over time add up to higher HDL-cholesterol and lower triglyceride levels.

One study in which middle-aged subjects with high blood cholesterol levels cycled for 30 to 60 minutes at 50 to 80 percent $\dot{V}O_2$max, burning 350 calories, showed that HDL-cholesterol remained elevated 9 percent for at least 48 hours postexercise, while triglycerides were still 15 percent below pre-exercise levels. No significant improvement in LDL-cholesterol, however, was measured, a finding consistent with the results of exercise training studies.

The largest acute increase in HDL-cholesterol occurs following unusually heavy exertion. For example, after a marathon race, HDL-cholesterol can increase 15 to 25 percent. Triglycerides drop sharply at the same time as the muscles use fats for fuel. In one study of 29 triathletes who finished the 1994 Hawaii Ironman World Championship, blood triglycerides dropped 39 percent.

# REFERENCES

Crouse, S.F., O'Brien, B.C., Rohack, J.J., et al. (1995). Changes in serum lipids and apolipoproteins after exercise in men with high cholesterol: Influence of intensity. *Journal of Applied Physiology, 79*, 279-286.

Ginsburg, G.S., Agil, A., O'Toole, M., Rimm, E., Douglas, P.S., & Rifai, N. (1996). Effects of a single bout of ultraendurance exercise on lipid levels and susceptibility of lipids to peroxidation in triathletes. *Journal of the American Medical Association, 276*, 221-225.

Grover, S.A., Coupal, L., & Hu, X-P. (1995). Identifying adults at increased risk of coronary disease: How well do the current cholesterol guidelines work? *Journal of the American Medical Association, 274*, 801-806.

Katzel, L.I., Bleecker, E.R., Colman, E.G., Rogus, E.M., Sorkin, J.D., & Goldberg, A.P. (1995). Effects of weight loss vs aerobic exercise training on risk factors for coronary disease in healthy, obese, middle-aged and older men. *Journal of the American Medical Association, 274*, 1915-1921.

Kokkinos, P.F., Holland, J.C., Narayan, P., Colleran, J.A., Dotson, C.O., & Papademetriou, V. (1995). Miles run per week and high-density lipoprotein cholesterol levels in healthy, middle-aged men: A dose-response relationship. *Archives of Internal Medicine, 155*, 415-420.

Pronk, N.P. (1993). Short term effects of exercise on plasma lipids and lipoproteins in humans. *Sports Medicine, 16*, 431-448.

Schwartz, R.S., Cain, K.C., Shuman, W.P., et al. (1992). Effect of intensive endurance training on lipoprotein profiles in young and older men. *Metabolism, 41*, 649-654.

Tsetsonis, N.V., Hardman, A.E., & Mastana, S.S. (1997). Acute effects of exercise on postprandial lipemia: A comparative study in trained and untrained middle-aged women. *American Journal of Clinical Nutrition, 65*, 525-533.

Walford, R.L., Harris, S.B., & Gunion, M.W. (1992). The calorically restricted low-fat nutrient-dense diet in Biosphere 2 significantly lowers blood glucose, total leukocyte count, cholesterol, and blood pressure in humans. *Proceedings of the National Academy of Sciences, 89*, 11533-11537.

Williams, P.T. (1996). High-density lipoprotein cholesterol and other risk factors for coronary heart disease in female runners. *New England Journal of Medicine, 334*, 1298-1303.

Wood, P.D. (1994). Physical activity, diet, and health: Independent and interactive effects. *Medicine and Science in Sports and Exercise, 26*, 838-843.

Chapter 14

# HIGH BLOOD PRESSURE

Given the high prevalence of a sedentary lifestyle among
U.S. residents, performance of moderate intensity, low resistance,
dynamic exercise, such as walking, cycling, dancing, and
gardening could play a valuable role in the prevention
of hypertension.

**National Health Blood Pressure Education Program,
National Heart, Lung, and Blood Institute**

Blood is carried from the heart to all of the body's tissues and organs in
vessels called arteries. Blood pressure is the force of the blood pushing
against the walls of those arteries. The heart beats about 60 to 75 times
each minute, and the blood pressure is at its greatest when the heart
contracts, pumping blood into the arteries. This is called systolic blood
pressure. When the heart is resting briefly between beats, the blood
pressure falls to a lower level, and is termed diastolic blood pressure (see
figure 14.1).

Both blood pressures are important, and they are usually presented
together, as in the expression 120/80 mmHg, with the first number
representing the systolic, and the second number the diastolic blood
pressure. According to the National High Blood Pressure Education
Program, blood pressures can be categorized as follows:

|  | **Systolic (mmHg)** | **Diastolic (mmHg)** |
|---|---|---|
| *Normal* | less than 130 | less than 85 |
| *High normal* | 130-139 | 85-89 |
| *High* | 140 and higher | 90 and higher |

**Blood Pressure**

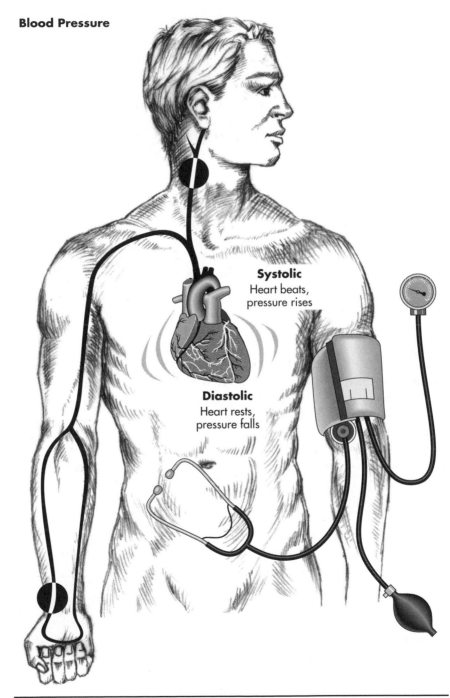

**Systolic**
Heart beats,
pressure rises

**Diastolic**
Heart rests,
pressure falls

FIGURE 14.1    Blood pressure is taken by sphygmomanometer while pulse is measured at the wrist or neck.

## Prevalence

More than 50 million people in the United States (about 20 percent) have high blood pressure, or hypertension, and nearly one-fourth don't even know they have it, according to the American Heart Association. Another 30 million adults have "high normal" blood pressures and are at high risk for developing high blood pressure later on in life. Two million new hypertensives are added each year to the pool of patients in the United States, so that by old age, about two-thirds of Americans have this disease.

The good news is that between 1960 and 1991, average U.S. systolic and diastolic blood pressures fell about 10 and 5 mmHg, respectively. Prevalence of high blood pressure has decreased for every age-sex-race subgroup except black men aged 50 and older.

## Health Problems

High blood pressure usually doesn't give early warning signs, and for this reason it is known as the "silent killer." High blood pressure kills more than 37,000 Americans each year and contributes to the deaths of more than 700,000, reports the National Center for Health Statistics. High blood pressure increases the risk for coronary heart disease and other forms of heart disease, stroke, and kidney failure.

According to the National Heart, Lung, and Blood Institute, when blood pressure is not detected and treated, it can

- cause the heart to get larger, which may lead to heart failure;
- cause small blisters (aneurisms) to form in the brain's blood vessels, which may cause a stroke;
- cause blood vessels in the kidney to narrow, which may cause kidney failure; and
- cause arteries throughout the body to "harden" faster, especially those in the heart, brain, and kidneys, which can cause a heart attack, stroke, or kidney failure.

High blood pressure also affects the brain. People with elevated blood pressure in middle age are more likely 25 years later to experience loss of cognitive abilities—memory, problem solving, concentration, and judgment. And this translates into a diminished capacity to function independently in old age.

Researchers from around the world have shown that in societies where salt and alcohol intakes are high, where potassium intake from fruits and vegetables is low, and where physical inactivity and obesity are the norm, hypertension is common. Risk of high blood pressure is also high among African Americans, people with a family history of hypertension, and those who are elderly.

## Treatment and Prevention

Controlled clinical trials have clearly shown that when people with hypertension faithfully use drugs to control their condition, death rates from heart disease and stroke decrease. Many people with hypertension, however, are not fully compliant in using their drugs, and as a result, fewer than one-third have their blood pressure under control. Many drug treatment regimens are expensive, and almost all blood pressure medications have some adverse side effects.

Although drugs play an important role in treatment, most hypertension experts now feel that prudent lifestyle habits lie at the foundation of both prevention and treatment of high blood pressure. The National Institutes of Health (NIH) has urged that Americans can do much to achieve normal blood pressures by following these recommendations:

• **Lose weight if overweight:** Studies have identified a strong relationship between body weight and blood pressure. Being overweight more than triples the risk of developing hypertension, with the risk climbing strongly with increasing body weight. Loss of excess body weight has been observed to be the most effective of all lifestyle strategies in normalizing the blood pressure. Losing just 5 to 10 pounds can decrease the diastolic blood pressure 5 mmHg, while a loss of 20 pounds or more doubles this improvement.

• **Reduce sodium intake to less than 2,300 mg (one teaspoon of salt) per day:** Most Western societies consume a diet that contains about one to two teaspoons of salt per day, with about 80 percent of this coming from processed foods, not the salt shaker. This is far in excess of what the body needs (which is only one-fifth of a teaspoon) and is much more than what our ancestors ingested. It is felt that when high salt intake is prolonged throughout the lifetime of a population, the majority will eventually experience high blood pressure. In many studies with hypertensive patients, lowering salt consumption by one-half teaspoon a day (e.g., from one and one-half to one teaspoon of salt) reduces systolic blood pressure by about 5 mmHg and diastolic blood pressure by about 2.5 mmHg. This effect is most likely to occur in elderly and African American patients. To keep sodium intake below 2,300 mg a day, nutrition experts urge that people learn to read food labels (to detect "hidden" salt in processed foods) and avoid foods high in sodium, choose more fresh fruits and vegetables, reduce use of salt during cooking while using more herbs and spices, avoid using the salt shaker on prepared foods, and limit the use of foods with visible salt on them.

• **Maintain adequate dietary potassium intake (fruits and vegetables):** Potassium, which is common in fresh fruits and vegetables, appears to help reduce blood pressure by increasing the amount of sodium that leaves the body in the urine. At least five to nine servings of fruits and vegetables are recommended each day to keep potassium intake at optimal levels.

• **Limit alcohol intake:** A large number of studies have shown that heavy alcohol consumption (three drinks or more a day on average) causes an increase in blood pressure. Among heavy drinkers, high blood pressure is four times more common than among those who avoid alcohol. And when people with hypertension who are heavy drinkers stop drinking, blood pressure falls. Most experts recommend less than two drinks a day to help avoid the risk of developing high blood pressure.

• **Exercise regularly:** As will be reviewed in the next section, regular aerobic exercise has now been shown to be a powerful tool in both preventing and treating high blood pressure.

The NIH urges that all Americans follow these preventive measures and that people with hypertension seek to control their high blood pressure with these lifestyle changes for at least three to six months before starting drug therapy. Even when drug therapy is necessary, weight loss, regular exercise, and other lifestyle modifications "should continue to be pursued vigorously," counsels the NIH.

According to experts at the NIH, lifestyle measures offer "multiple benefits at little cost and with minimal risk. Even when not adequate in themselves to control hypertension, they may reduce the number and doses of antihypertensive medications needed to manage the condition."

## EXERCISE-HEALTH CONNECTION

When a person walks briskly, cycles, jogs, swims, or engages in other aerobic activities, the blood pressure rises strongly. For example, during intense aerobic exercise the systolic blood pressure can climb from a resting level of 110 to 120 mmHg to 150 to 200 mmHg. Interestingly, if the blood pressure surges too steeply (i.e., well above 200 mmHg) during a standardized exercise test, risk of future hypertension or heart disease is unusually high, even in subjects with normal resting blood pressures.

Soon after the aerobic session is over, the blood pressure falls below normal levels, an effect that can last for at least 30 to 120 minutes. The effect is especially dramatic in hypertensive patients. In a study conducted by Dr. Patricia Rueckert of the University of Wisconsin Medical School on 18 patients with high blood pressure, 45 minutes of brisk treadmill walking lowered the blood pressure below resting levels for at least two hours of recovery. The acute decrease in blood pressure was related to a widening and relaxation of the blood vessels.

Over time, as the exercise is repeated, growing evidence suggests that a long-lasting reduction in resting blood pressure can be experienced. In other words, exercise training may lower the blood pressure through the beneficial and additive effects of regular bouts of physical activity.

---

### *If I exercise regularly, can I prevent high blood pressure or cure it if I have it?*

The answer to both these questions is yes, with researchers now concluding that exercise is a potent weapon against high blood pressure.

---

With regard to prevention, several major studies have shown that inactive and unfit individuals have a 20- to 50-percent increased risk of developing hypertension compared to their more physically active peers. In a 6- to 10-year study of 15,000 Harvard male alumni, for example, those who did not engage in vigorous sport and physical activity were at 35 percent greater risk of becoming hypertensive than those who were active. In a study at the Cooper Institute for Aerobics Research, physically unfit individuals were found to be 52 percent more likely to develop high blood pressure than those who were physically fit (as measured on a treadmill).

Exercise has a strong effect in treating high blood pressure. The American College of Sports Medicine (ACSM) and other reviewers have concluded that people with mild hypertension can expect systolic and diastolic blood pressures to fall an average of 8 to 10 mmHg and 6 to 10 mmHg, respectively, in response to regular aerobic exercise. This benefit is independent of changes in body weight or diet (which can result in greater reductions). Even for people with normal resting blood pressures, exercise training can be expected to lower the systolic and diastolic blood pressures by an average of 4 mmHg and 3 mmHg, respectively.

The improvement in blood pressure with exercise training may extend to patients with severe hypertension, but few studies exist to confirm this. Dr. Peter Kokkinos of the Veterans Affairs Medical Center in Washington, D.C., studied the effects of 16 to 32 weeks of moderate exercise (stationary cycling, three times a week, 20 to 60 minutes a session at 60 to 80 percent of maximum heart rate) on the blood pressures of African American men with severe hypertension. As a safety precaution, prior to initiating exercise training, diastolic blood pressures were reduced at least 10 mmHg with medication.

As shown in figure 14.2, exercise subjects experienced strong decreases in blood pressure after 16 weeks. Exercise training continued for an additional 16 weeks, and doses of medication were reduced in 71 percent of the exercise subjects, but none of the controls. Concluded Dr. Kokkinos, "Our results show that severe hypertension can be managed more effectively with a combination of drug therapy and regular, moderately intense exercise. Most important, medications necessary to control blood pressure without exercise can be curtailed substantially as patients continue exercising."

The data are convincing enough to prompt this statement by experts writing the first Surgeon General's report on physical activity and health: "Regular physical activity prevents or delays the development

**Effects of Exercise in African American Men With Severe Hypertension**
*16 weeks of cycling, 20–60 minutes/session, 60%–80% maximum heart rate*

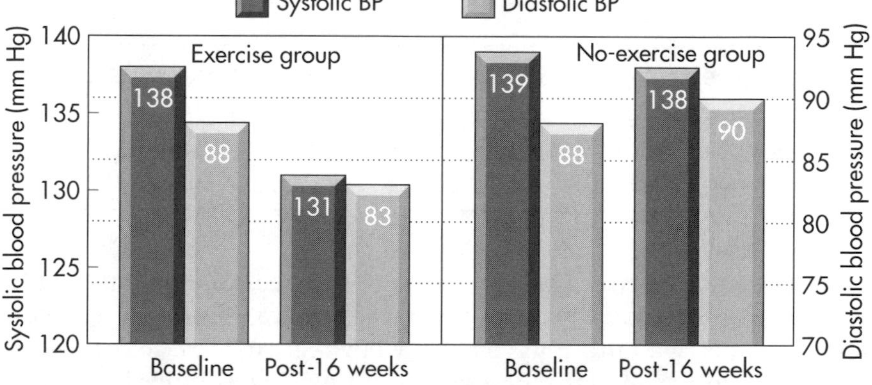

FIGURE 14.2   Regular exercise reduced blood pressure in African American men with severe hypertension.

of high blood pressure, and exercise reduces blood pressure in people with hypertension."

---

### How long do I have to exercise before I see an improvement in my resting blood pressure?

Most studies show that exercise training acts quickly to improve blood pressure among people with hypertension, with most of the effect taking place within the first few weeks. Further reductions in blood pressure may occur if the exercise training is maintained for more than three months.

---

Dr. Michael Kelemen, for example, reported in the *Journal of the American Medical Association* the results from a study in which people with hypertension exercised aerobically three times a week for 10 weeks while taking either a diuretic or beta-blocker (i.e., hypertensive drugs) or a placebo (a pill with no drug in it). Exercise alone without drugs resulted in an impressive 8 mmHg drop in the diastolic blood pressure within the first month, with drug therapy adding a little extra benefit. Interestingly, most of the improvement in blood pressure occurred during the first week, with some additional progress measured as the training continued.

Soon after a person stops exercise training, however, blood pressure returns to its initial untrained level. In other words, the blood pressure-lowering effect of exercise training depends on a regular schedule of activity.

---

### What type of exercise works best in lowering blood pressure?

The ACSM has established that effective lowering of blood pressure can be achieved with moderate-intensity aerobic exercise conducted three to five times a week for 20 to 60 minutes per session.

---

The aerobic exercise program does not have to be too demanding to improve resting blood pressure. In fact, moderate-intensity exercise such as brisk walking may have an even greater blood pressure-lowering effect than higher-intensity training (like running) for some people. The important exercise criterion is frequency: Near-daily activity helps the body experience, on a regular basis, the beneficial effects of exercise in lowering blood pressure.

The ACSM does not recommend weight training as the only form of exercise for people who have hypertension. Weight training does not appear to be as effective in lowering blood pressure as aerobic exercise, although it is an excellent way to increase muscular strength and is recommended for overall physical fitness. Experts recommend, however, that people with hypertension avoid maximal lifts, instead emphasizing weight lifts that they can perform for 10 to 15 repetitions.

---

### How does regular exercise lower the blood pressure?

Although researchers are still studying the causes, exercise does appear to relax the blood vessels. Both acute and chronic changes may occur in nerve activity, hormone receptors, and the local production of certain chemicals.

---

As discussed earlier in this chapter, each exercise session relaxes the blood vessels, causing a postexercise decrease in blood pressure. Over time, exercise may "loosen up" the blood vessels a bit, lowering the resting blood pressure in much the same way that widening a water pipe lowers water pressure.

The blood vessels may relax after each exercise session because of body-warming effects, local production of certain chemicals (e.g., lactic acid and nitric oxide), decreases in nerve activity, and changes in certain hormones and their receptors. As the exercise is repeated regularly, all of these acute effects may create a chronic lowering of the blood pressure.

---

### Is it safe for people with high blood pressure to exercise?

Yes, but those with severe hypertension should first use medication to help bring their blood pressures under better control.

---

Present studies do not support the concern that people with high blood pressure are at increased risk for sudden death during exercise. However, for people with blood pressure greater than 180/110 mmHg, most experts recommend the use of medication to lower the blood pressure prior to starting an exercise program. Some individuals with enlarged hearts (from the hypertension) should keep the intensity of exercise at moderate levels to prevent further damage.

People with high blood pressure have been shown to be less fit (about 30 percent) than those with normal blood pressures. Thus regular aerobic exercise is critical in order for hypertensive patients to improve physical fitness and life quality and to lower risk for heart disease. Dr. Steven Blair of the Cooper Institute for Aerobics Research has demonstrated in a large study of more than 32,000 men and women that death rates are lower in highly fit people, even if their blood pressures are high, than in those with low aerobic fitness and normal blood pressures.

Previously, people with high blood pressure were counseled not to engage in weight training because of fears of an unusually high blood pressure response. Extremely high blood pressures have been measured in weight lifters during maximal lifts. In circuit weight training, however, elevations in blood pressure are modest because people lift moderate loads (30 to 50 percent of maximum) 10 to 15 times, with short rest intervals, at 10 to 12 different stations. While intensive weight training should be avoided, circuit weight training is recommended as a component of a well-rounded exercise program that includes aerobic activities.

# REFERENCES

American College of Sports Medicine. (1993). Physical activity, physical fitness and hypertension. *Medicine and Science in Sports and Exercise, 25*, i-x.

Blair, S.N., Kampert, J.B., Kohl, H.W., et al. (1996). Influences of cardiorespiratory fitness and other precursors on cardiovascular disease and all-cause mortality in men and women. *Journal of the American Medical Association, 276*, 205-210.

Burt, V.L., Cutler, J.A., Higgins, M., Horan, M.J., Labarthe, D., Whelton, P., Brown, C., & Roccella, E.J. (1995). Trends in the prevalence, awareness, treatment, and control of hypertension in the adult US population: Data from the Health Examination Surveys, 1960 to 1991. *Hypertension, 26*, 60-69.

DiCarlo, S.E., Collins, H.L., Howard, M.G., Chen, C-Y., Scislo, T.J., & Patil, R.D. (1994). Postexertional hypotension: A brief review. *Sports Medicine, Training, and Rehabilitation, 5*, 17-27.

Kelemen, M.H., Effron, M.B., Valenti, S.A., & Stewart, K.J. (1990). Exercise training combined with antihypertensive drug therapy: Effects on lipids, blood pressure, and left ventricular mass. *Journal of the American Medical Association, 263*, 2766-2771.

Kelley, G. (1995). Effects of weight lifting on resting blood pressure: A meta-analysis. *Sports Medicine, Training, and Rehabilitation, 6*, 61-69.

Kelley, G., & Tran, Z.V. (1995). Aerobic exercise and normotensive adults: A meta-analysis. *Medicine and Science in Sports and Exercise, 27*, 1371-1377.

Kokkinos, P.F., Narayan, P., Colleran, J.A., Pittaras, A., Notargiacomo, A., Reda, D., & Papademetriou, V. (1995). Effects of regular exercise on blood pressure and left ventricular hypertrophy in African-American men with severe hypertension. *New England Journal of Medicine, 333,* 1462-1467.

Launer, L.J., Masaki, K., Petrovitch, H., Foley, D., & Havlik, R.J. (1995). The association between midlife blood pressure levels and late-life cognitive function: The Honolulu-Asia aging study. *Journal of the American Medical Association, 274,* 1846-1851.

Lim, P.O., MacFadyen, R.J., Clarkson, P.B., & MacDonald, T.M. (1996). Impaired exercise tolerance in hypertensive patients. *Annals of Internal Medicine, 124* (1 Part 1), 41-55.

Mundal, R., Kjeldsen, S.E., Sandvik, L., Erikssen, G., Thaulow, E., & Erikssen, J. (1996). Exercise blood pressure predicts mortality from myocardial infarction. *Hypertension, 27* (Part 1), 324-329.

National High Blood Pressure Education Program. (1993). *The fifth report of the joint national committee on detecction, evaluation, and treatment of high blood pressure.* NHLBI, NIH, NIH Publication No. 93-1088. Bethesda, MD: National Institutes of Health.

Rueckert, P.A., Slane, P.R., Lillis, D.L., & Hanson, P. (1996). Hemodynamic patterns and duration of post-dynamic exercise hypotension in hypertensive humans. *Medicine and Science in Sports and Exercise, 28,* 24-32.

U.S. Department of Health and Human Services. (1996). *Physical activity and health: A report of the Surgeon General.* Atlanta: U.S. Department of Health and Human Services, Centers for Disease Control and Prevention, National Center for Chronic Disease Prevention and Health Promotion.

# Chapter 15

# NUTRITIONAL HABITS

People who are inactive or trying to lose weight may eat little food and have difficulty meeting their nutrient needs in a satisfying diet. Nearly all Americans need to be more active, because a sedentary lifestyle is unhealthy. Increasing the energy spent in daily activities helps to maintain health and allows people to eat a nutritious and enjoyable diet.

**The United States Department of Agriculture**

If you start a regular exercise program, will you also feel like eating better? Stated another way, will exercise help you bring your eating habits under good control? I have conducted several exercise training studies in which I assigned women to a brisk walking group or a nonwalking control group for 12 to 15 weeks and carefully monitored their diets for change. What do you think I found? We'll explore the answer later in this chapter.

## THE PRUDENT DIET

Americans tend to eat too much energy in the form of fat, especially the hard saturated fat common in animal products. They also have diets too low in starch and fiber, found in plant foods like whole grains, fruits, and vegetables. Such diets explain why Americans have high rates of obesity, heart disease, high blood pressure, stroke, diabetes, and some forms of cancer.

It should be noted that diseases caused by vitamin and mineral deficiencies are rare in this country and other developed nations. Very few people die anymore from scurvy (vitamin C deficiency), pellagra (niacin deficiency), or beriberi (riboflavin deficiency).

For all individuals, whether physically active or inactive, a "prudent diet" is recommended for general health and prevention of disease.

Figure 15.1 summarizes the proportion of total energy intake recommended for carbohydrate (55 percent), fat (30 percent), and protein (15 percent). This type of diet is advocated for fitness enthusiasts (those exercising three to five days per week, 20 to 30 minutes per session) and nearly all athletes, including those in most individual, dual, and team sports and power events (weight lifting, track and field). For the competitive endurance athlete (who trains more than 90 minutes a day in such sports as running, swimming, and cycling), several adaptations beyond the prudent diet are beneficial, including a higher percentage of carbohydrate, less fat, and more water. (Sport nutrition principles will be reviewed later in this chapter.)

**The Prudent Diet: Proportion of Calories as Carbohydrate, Fat, Protein**

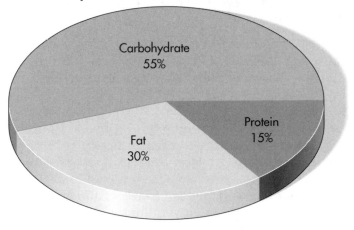

FIGURE 15.1   The prudent diet is recommended for all Americans and fitness enthusiasts.

In this chapter, the prudent diet will be defined as that conforming to the 1995 *Nutrition and Your Health: Dietary Guidelines for Americans* of the U.S. Department of Agriculture (USDA). There are seven major dietary guidelines according to the USDA:

**1. Eat a variety of foods.** More than 40 different nutrients classified into six groups (protein, carbohydrate, fat, vitamin, mineral, and water) are needed for good health. These nutrients should come from a variety of foods, not from a few highly fortified foods or supplements. No single food can supply all of them in the amounts needed. Supplements of some nutrients taken regularly in large amounts can be harmful, due to direct toxicity or interference with the absorption of other nutrients. Some people use supplements to try to "cover up" their poor dietary habits—something that cannot be done with pills and capsules. As a general rule, most Americans don't need supplements for good health.

Diet variety is probably the single most important nutrition principle. The USDA urges that all people try to follow the recommendations of the "Food Guide Pyramid," consuming at least the lower number of servings suggested from each food group per day (see figure 15.2). Grains and cereals should form the basis of each meal, supplemented with liberal servings of vegetables and fruit and low-fat servings of dairy and meat products. Typical serving sizes are one slice of bread or one-half cup of pasta; one-half cup of cooked vegetables; one medium apple, banana, or other fruit; one cup of milk or yogurt; and two to three ounces of cooked lean meat, poultry, or fish.

Unfortunately, Americans fall short of following the diet variety outlined in the Food Pyramid. According to the USDA, fewer than one-third of American adults consume five or more servings of fruits and vegetables each day, and the intake of nutrient-packed dark green and deep yellow vegetables is much lower than recommended. This is disturbing, because many experts feel that a high fruit and vegetable intake is one of the best ways to keep cancer at bay.

**2. Balance the food eaten with physical activity. Maintain or improve weight.** Being overweight is common in the United States (33 percent of adults and 20 percent of adolescents) and is linked with high blood pressure, heart disease, stroke, diabetes, certain cancers, arthritis, and other types of illness. One can maintain a healthy weight by being physically active and consuming a variety of foods low in calories and fat, such as fruits, vegetables, whole grains, nonfat dairy products, and baked fish or poultry.

Caloric intake among Americans is about 6 percent higher than it was two decades ago (now about 2,500 and 1,600 calories per day for men and women, respectively). At the same time, according to the Surgeon General, more than 60 percent of American adults are not regularly physically active. In fact, 25 percent of all adults are not active at all. It is obvious that the increase in prevalence of obesity has occurred because many people eat more calories than they expend.

It should be noted that the 1995 USDA Dietary Guidelines for Americans for the first time included physical activity as a key ingredient in the recommendations. In 1990 the guideline read "Maintain healthy weight"; in 1995 this was changed to "Balance the food you eat with physical activity; maintain or improve your weight."

**3. Choose a diet with plenty of grain products, vegetables, and fruits.** As outlined under guideline #1, more servings of grain products should be eaten at each meal than for any other type of food; the next

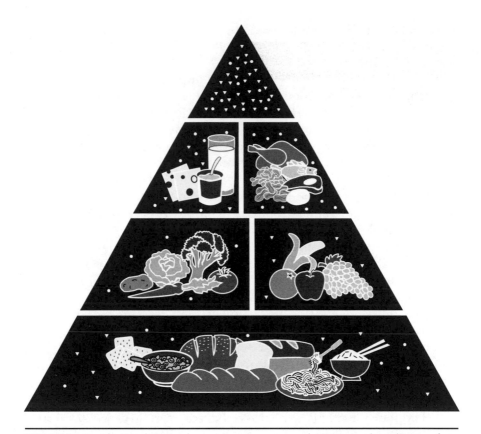

**FIGURE 15.2**  The Food Pyramid urges Americans to emphasize cereals and grains, fruits and vegetables in their diet.

highest number of servings should be of fruits and vegetables. Grains (e.g., pasta, rice, wheat, cereals) should form the center of most meals. When one chooses more whole-grain products, fruits, and vegetables, carbohydrate and fiber intake will increase while fat and cholesterol intake decrease.

A high dietary fiber intake has been associated with a lower risk of colon cancer and is an important component of the diet used to help control blood glucose levels in diabetics. People who include a high number of servings of vegetables, fruits, and whole grains tend to have less heart disease and cancer than those who tend to avoid these foods.

Most authorities recommend that at least 55 percent of calories come from carbohydrate. For an individual eating 2,000 calories a day, this would be 1,100 calories or 275 grams of carbohydrate (1,100 ÷ 4, the number of calories per gram of carbohydrate). The average American male adult consumes an average of only 49 percent of calories from carbohydrate, with females averaging 52 percent. And much of this carbohydrate is in the form of processed sugar instead of the preferable starch (also called complex carbohydrate).

The National Cancer Institute recommends that people eat 20 to 30 grams of dietary fiber each day. Dietary fiber is only found in plant foods and is especially abundant in legumes (7 grams per half cup), nuts and seeds (4 to 9 grams per half cup), whole grains (3 to 5 grams per cup), fresh fruits (2 to 9 grams per cup), and vegetables (2 to 5 grams per cup). American females average only 14, and males, 19 grams of dietary fiber a day in their diets, well below the recommended range.

**4. Choose a diet low in fat, saturated fat, and cholesterol.** According to the National Research Council, "A large and convincing body of evidence from studies in humans and laboratory animals shows that diets low in saturated fatty acids and cholesterol are associated with low risk and rates of cardiovascular disease." High-fat diets have also been related to some types of cancer and are a major factor explaining human obesity.

Total dietary fat intake should be less than 30 percent of the calories a person consumes, with saturated fat less than 10 percent of calories. For example, at 2,000 calories per day, the suggested upper limit for total fat is 600 calories (2,000 × 0.30). This is equal to 67 grams of fat (600 ÷ 9, the number of calories each gram of fat provides). For saturated fat, no more than 200 out of 2,000 calories should be ingested, which amounts to 22 grams (200 ÷ 9). American adult males average 34 percent total calories as fat, and females, 33 percent. For saturated fat, both males and females adults average 11 percent in their diets. Only one-third of Americans keep their intake under 30 percent of total energy intake.

The fats in animal products (dairy products and meats) are the main sources of saturated fat in most diets, with tropical oils (e.g., palm oils) and hydrogenated fats (e.g., stick margarines) providing smaller amounts.

Cholesterol intake should be below 300 milligrams per day. At 212 milligrams per day, the average intake by women is below this level. However, at 334 milligrams per day, the average intake by men exceeds the recommended level. Animal products are the source of all dietary cholesterol—egg yolks being one of the richest sources, with each one containing about 220 milligrams of cholesterol. In general, it is recommended that one choose low-fat or fat-free dairy products, consume lean cuts of meat, and learn to prepare foods with low amounts of fat.

**5. Choose a diet moderate in sugars.** Sugars and many foods that contain them in large amounts (e.g., soft drinks, desserts) supply calories but are limited in nutrients. Sugars also promote tooth decay. Thus they should be used in moderation by most healthy people and more sparingly by people with low calorie needs. Intake of sugar has not been associated with increased risk of heart disease, cancer, or diabetes, however.

**6. Choose a diet moderate in salt and sodium.** Table salt is 40 percent sodium, with one teaspoon of salt containing 2,000 milligrams of sodium. Many health experts recommend less than 3,000 milligrams of sodium per day (less than one and one-half teaspoons of salt) to lower the risk of developing high blood pressure. Most people eat more salt and sodium than they need, averaging 4,000 to 6,000 milligrams of sodium a day. The richest sources of sodium are sauces, salad dressings, cheeses, processed meats, soups, and grain-cereal products.

**7. If you drink alcoholic beverages, do so in moderation.** Alcoholic beverages supply calories but few or no nutrients. Drinking them has no net health benefit, is linked with many health problems, is the cause of many accidents, is associated with many violent crimes, and can lead to addiction. While it is true that moderate amounts of alcohol lower risk of coronary heart disease, the risk of several forms of cancer is increased.

If adults elect to drink alcoholic beverages, they should consume them in moderate amounts, defined as no more than two drinks a day for men and one drink a day for women. One drink is defined as 12 ounces of regular beer, 5 ounces of wine, and 1.5 ounces of distilled spirits (80 proof), each of which contains 0.5 ounces of pure ethanol. The National Institute on Alcohol Abuse and Alcoholism reports that over 15 million Americans are either alcoholics or alcohol abusers.

Put simply, these guidelines stress the need for many Americans to eat more plant foods (fruits, vegetables, and whole grains) while eating less high-fat dairy products and meats. These guidelines call for moderation—avoiding extremes in diet. Moderate intake of visible fats and oils, sugars, salt, and alcoholic beverages (if used at all) is emphasized.

## EXERCISE-HEALTH CONNECTION

The average American not only exercises less than recommended, but also falls short of conforming to the USDA Dietary Guidelines for Americans. As will be pointed out in the next section, even athletes have been found to eat more fat and less carbohydrate than recommended for their activity levels.

Two types of studies are available in answering this important question: comparisons of the diets of athletes and nonathletes, or physically active and inactive people; and exercise training studies, in which inactive people are assigned to exercise and control groups to determine whether people initiating exercise spontaneously improve the quality of their diets.

---

### What does exercise have to do with the kind of food I eat?

Most experts feel that exercise in and of itself has a minor influence on the quality of the diet. However, with increasing amounts of exercise, people tend to eat more, increasing their overall intake of essential vitamins and minerals.

---

Many reports on the diets of athletes and nonathletes are available. In general, most researchers have found that athletes, especially those in endurance sports like running and cycling, have slightly healthier diets than nonathletes. The contrast is more impressive for the most serious athletes. As Dr. Leonard Wankel of the University of Alberta in Canada has emphasized, "The positive association of physical activity involvement and good nutritional practices is most clearly evident in selected groups like serious runners."

Although there are notable exceptions, many athletes feel that a good diet gives them a competitive edge and therefore try to keep carbohydrate intake higher and fat intake lower than normal. It is interesting, however, that most groups of athletes have been found to be eating more fat and less carbohydrate than recommended for their athletic endeavors.

What about people who exercise regularly but are not competitive athletes? Most studies that have compared physically active and inactive people have shown that indeed, people who exercise regularly do have better diets. Figure 15.3 summarizes the results of a large study of 30,000 Americans conducted by the Centers for Disease Control and Prevention. Consumption of 13 high-fat food items and participation in physical activities were surveyed. A "fat intake score" was developed based on how frequently people ate such foods as hot dogs, lunch meats, bacon, sausage, hamburgers, cheeseburgers, meat loaf, fried chicken, cheese, butter, whole milk, etc. As shown in figure 15.3, people who exercised intensely on a regular basis had the lowest odds of being rated high-fat consumers, while physically inactive people were found to be most likely to eat high-fat foods on a frequent basis.

One problem with the group comparison studies is that researchers are unable to sort out why serious exercisers have diets superior to those of their sedentary peers. Is it because the exercise spontaneously prompts them to eat better? Or could it be that people motivated enough to exercise regularly also are disciplined enough to choose healthy foods?

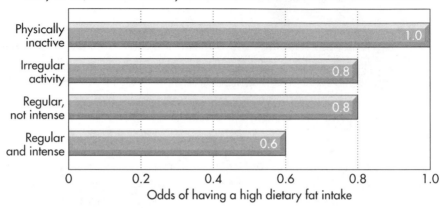

**Relationship Between Physical Activity and Dietary Fat Intake**
*Study of 30,000 Americans by the Centers for Disease Control and Prevention*

FIGURE 15.3    In this national study, the odds of a high fat intake was lowest among those who exercised.

One way of providing answers to these questions is to randomly divide sedentary subjects into exercise and nonexercise groups and then follow them for several months, measuring their diets along the way to see if quality changes. This is a difficult type of study to conduct, but most investigators have concluded that moderate exercise (e.g., brisk walking three to five days a week for 20 to 45 minutes a session) is an insufficient stimulus to cause people to make meaningful changes in the quality of their diets.

It is interesting, however, that as the exercise continues and is increased to higher levels, people start to eat more. Nutritionists feel that this is one of the chief benefits of regular and vigorous or long-duration (>45 minutes per day) exercise: People take in more food and energy, increasing their chances of getting all of the recommended amounts of vitamins and minerals.

Figure 15.4 shows the results of an interesting study of physically fit and unfit elderly women (average age, 73 years). Often as people grow older, they become more and more sedentary. To avoid weight gain, they eat less and less food, increasing the risk of low nutrient intake. In this study, the diets of very active elderly women who were exercising more than one hour a day were compared to those who were largely sedentary. Notice that when energy and nutrient intake was adjusted for body weight (because the sedentary women were heavier), the physically fit elderly women consumed 54 percent more energy, which led to a greater intake of nearly every vitamin and mineral measured.

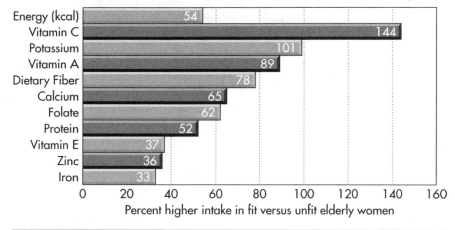

**Nutrient Intake in Physically Fit and Unfit Elderly Women**
*Percent difference in nutrient intake per kilogram of body weight*

FIGURE 15.4   Physically fit elderly women eat more, improving nutrient intake into the body.

### Should the diets of exercisers be any different from the diets of people who don't exercise?

Most experts emphasize an increase in total energy intake, especially from carbohydrates, with a liberal supply of fluids to replace sweat loss. For the vast majority of athletes, vitamin and mineral supplements are not needed if the diet is varied and balanced.

As time spent in aerobic-type exercise (running, swimming, bicycling, aerobic dance, etc.) increases, several changes in the diet are recommended:

- Increase in energy intake
- Increase in the percentage of calories coming from carbohydrate
- Increase in fluid intake

For highly active individuals, energy intake must increase (unless weight loss is the desired goal). At the same time, the proportion of fat in the diet should decrease as the amount of dietary carbohydrate increases. Some of the best sources of carbohydrate include cereals, dried fruits, breads, and pasta. Table 15.1 summarizes the recommended changes in energy, carbohydrate, and fat.

## TABLE 15.1
### The Energy Supply and Quality of Diet Recommended for People Who Exercise

| | Calories* | | % of Total Energy Intake | | |
|---|---|---|---|---|---|
| | Males | Females | Carbohydrate | Fat | Protein |
| Average American | 2,500 | 1,600 | 51 | 33 | 16 |
| Fitness enthusiasts | 2,900 | 2,000 | 55 | 30 | 15 |
| Endurance athletes | 3,500 | 2,600 | 60-70 | 15-25 | 15 |
| Team/power athletes | 4,000 | 3,000 | 55 | 30 | 15 |

* Energy intake can vary widely depending on body size and amount of exercise.

A high-carbohydrate diet is probably the most important nutritional principle for people who exercise. During exercise, the body prefers to use carbohydrate to supply energy to the working muscles. When the body carbohydrate stores drop too low, the ability to exercise hard falls, and one can feel stale and tired.

To increase carbohydrate and lower fat intake, most experts recommend that athletes consume less visible fats (margarine, oil, salad dressing, mayonnaise, etc.), less high-fat dairy products (most cheeses, whole milk, butter, cream cheese, etc.), less high-fat meats (fried meats, bacon, corned beef, ground beef, ham, sausages, processed meats, etc.), and more grain products (pasta, bagels, breads, brown rice, cereals, etc.), tubers (potatoes, yams), legumes (kidney beans, pinto beans, etc.), dried fruits (raisins, dates, etc.), fresh fruits, and fresh vegetables.

Probably the second most important dietary principle for individuals who exercise is to drink large quantities of water. As little as a three-pound drop in body weight due to water loss from sweating (which can happen within one hour, especially on hot, humid days) decreases the ability to exercise. Various studies have shown that the thirst desire of the exercising individual lags behind actual body needs. So before, during, and after an exercise bout, people should drink plenty of fluids, even beyond what they may feel like drinking. A plan recommended by some sports medicine experts is to drink two cups of water immediately before the exercise bout, one cup every 15 minutes during the exercise session, and then two more cups after the session.

Most studies show that the intake of protein and major vitamins and minerals is above recommended dietary intake levels in people who exercise. Physically active people tend to be at an advantage because they eat more than sedentary people, supplying their bodies with higher quantities of vitamins, minerals, and protein. The American Dietetic Association, in its publication *Nutrition for Physical Fitness and Athletic Performance for Adults*, has stated that heavy endurance exercise "may increase the need for some vitamins and minerals, but this can easily be met by consuming a balanced diet in accordance with the extra caloric requirement."

---

### I've heard that bodybuilders and other athletes should eat more protein to build their muscles. Is that true?

Yes, it is true that athletes need more protein than those who avoid exercise. However, the extra protein can be easily obtained from the traditional food supply without supplements.

---

Interest in the effect of dietary protein on athletic performance dates back to the days of the ancient Greeks and Romans. Athletes in those days ate meat-rich diets in the belief that they would achieve the strength of the consumed animal. Many strength athletes today use protein supplements because they feel that the extra protein will enhance gains in muscle size.

The average American diet has more than enough protein to meet the needs of all types of exercise programs, even weightlifting. The average inactive person has been advised to consume about 50 to 60 grams of protein a day, an amount that most easily achieve. In fact, the average American male eats close to 100 grams of protein a day (females get 65 grams per day). While research has established that some weight trainers may need an extra 25 to 50 grams of protein a day during active muscle-building phases, this is easily obtained in the diet without the use of protein supplements. Put another way, the average American male already eats the amount of protein needed by active weight trainers!

# REFERENCES

ADA Reports. (1993). Position of the American Dietetic Association and the Canadian Dietetic Association: Nutrition for physical fitness and athletic performance for adults. *Journal of the American Dietetic Association, 93*, 691-696.

Butterworth, D.E., Nieman, D.C., Perkins, R., Warren, B.J., & Dotson, R.G. (1993). Exercise training and nutrient intake in elderly women. *Journal of the American Dietetic Association, 93*, 653-657.

Butterworth, D.E., Nieman, D.C., Underwood, B.C., & Lindsted, K.D. (1994). The relationship between cardiorespiratory fitness, physical activity, and dietary quality. *International Journal of Sport Nutrition, 4,* 289-298.

Cleveland, L.E., Goldman, J.D., & Borrud, L.G. (1996). *Data tables: Results from USDA's 1994 Continuing Survey of Food Intakes by Individuals and 1994 Diet and Health Knowledge Survey.* Riverdale, MD: U.S. Department of Agriculture, Agricultural Research Service, Beltsville Human Nutrition Research Center, Food Surveys Research Group.

Federation of American Societies for Experimental Biology, Life Sciences Research Office. (1995). *Third report on nutrition monitoring in the United States: Executive summary.* Washington, DC: U.S. Government Printing Office.

Millard-Stafford, M., Rosskopf, L.B., Snow, T.K., & Hinson, B.T. (1997). Water versus carbohydrate-electrolyte ingestion before and during a 15-km run in the heat. *International Journal of Sport Nutrition, 7,* 26-38.

Nieman, D.C. (1995). *Fitness and sports medicine: A health-related approach.* Mountain View, CA: Mayfield.

Nieman, D.C., Onasch, L.M., & Lee, J.W. (1990). The effects of moderate exercise training on nutrient intake in mildly obese women. *Journal of the American Dietetic Association, 90,* 1557-1562.

Shephard, R.J. (1989). Exercise and lifestyle change. *British Journal of Sports Medicine, 23,* 11-22.

Simoes, E.J., Byers, T., Coates, R.J., Serdula, M.K., Mokdad, A.H., & Health, G.W. (1995). The association between leisure-time physical activity and dietary fat in American adults. *American Journal of Public Health, 85,* 240-244.

U.S. Department of Agriculture. (1995). *Nutrition and your health: Dietary guidelines for Americans* (Home and Garden Bulletin No. 232). Washington, DC: U.S. Department of Agriculture.

Wankel, L.M., & Sefton, J.M. (1994). Physical activity and other lifestyle behaviors. In C. Bouchard, R.J. Shephard, & T. Stephens (Eds.), *Physical activity, fitness, and health: International proceedings and consensus statement.* Champaign, IL: Human Kinetics.

Williams, M. (1997, January-February). The gospel truth about dietary supplements. *ACSM's Health and Fitness Journal,* 24-29.

# Chapter 16

# SLEEP

The sleep of a laborer is sweet, whether he eats little or much, but
the abundance of a rich man permits him no sleep.

Ecclesiastes 5:12

A common belief among many fitness enthusiasts is that regular exercise helps them sleep better. James Fixx, in his best seller *The Complete
Book of Running,* which helped fuel the fitness boom of the 1980s, wrote,
"After a run you'll feel refreshed. You'll have more energy, more zest.
. . . You'll sleep more soundly, lose weight if you need to, and feel better
than you have in years." This belief will be explored for its accuracy later
in the chapter. First, just what is this thing called sleep?

## SLEEP DISORDERS

Medical textbooks define sleep as an "unconsciousness from which the
person can be aroused by sensory or other stimuli." In other words, it is
unlike coma, which is "unconsciousness from which the person cannot
be aroused." If recent data are any indication, many Americans may
prefer a few bouts of coma to one of insomnia, now among the most
prevalent health complaints.

Insomnia is defined by the National Institutes of Health as "the
perception or complaint of inadequate or poor-quality sleep." Characteristics of insomnia include

- difficulty falling asleep,
- waking up frequently during the night with difficulty returning to
  sleep,
- waking up too early in the morning, and
- unrefreshing sleep.

According to the Better Sleep Council, a nonprofit organization established in 1978 and recognized as one of the leading sleep educators in the United States and Canada, "Sleep problems have become a modern epidemic that is taking an enormous toll on our bodies and minds. Desperately trying to fit more into the hours of the day, many people are stealing extra hours from the night."

Yet often, even those who want to sleep more can't because the stress of the day wreaks havoc on the brain during the night. "The frantic pace of modern society is leaving more Americans awake when they shouldn't be," says Dr. Allan Pack, medical director of the National Sleep Foundation. "One of every five Americans may be living in a twilight zone of sleep deprivation," adds the Better Sleep Council, "that undermines their health, sabotages their productivity, blackens their mood, clouds their judgment and increases their risk of accidents."

According to a report issued by the National Commission on Sleep Disorders Research, as many as 80 million Americans have serious, incapacitating sleep problems, 20 to 40 percent have insomnia, and nearly half of older adults say they can't get a solid night's rest. The vast majority of Americans fail to understand what to do about poor sleep and the consequences.

Sleep loss and sleep disturbances are thought to play a major role in 200,000 to 400,000 automobile accidents each year, with as many as 13 percent of accident-related fatalities caused by falling asleep at the wheel. The loss of one hour's sleep when most Americans "spring forward" in April to daylight saving time causes an average increase of 7 to 8 percent in traffic accidents. Conversely, the switch back to standard time in the fall causes a 7 to 8 percent decrease.

People with chronic insomnia have a diminished ability to concentrate, memory problems, trouble in carrying out daily tasks, and difficulty in working with and getting along with other people. Poor sleep can result in fatigue, increasing the opportunity for human error and accidents.

Shift workers account for 20 percent of the U.S. work force and are two to five times more likely to fall asleep on the job than day workers, while exhibiting more stress and irritability and experiencing more heart disease and stomach/intestinal ailments. British researchers and a team at Brigham and Women's Hospital and Harvard Medical School in Boston studied 24 healthy adults who rotated their sleep patterns so that they went to bed four hours later every night for several weeks, creating a kind of jet lag. The study showed that when the sleep schedule was altered, mood deteriorated. Dr. Diane Boivin, who headed up the study, says that "shift workers may experience more anxiety and depression, partly because they are out of sync with their biological clocks."

Interestingly, sleep duration is related to length of life. In one large study of a million Americans, those aged 45 years or older who reported sleeping more than 10 hours per night or fewer than 5 hours per night had higher death rates during follow-up than those sleeping about 7 hours a night.

# SLEEP CYCLES

A night's sleep consists of four or five cycles, each of which progresses through several stages. Each stage produces specific brain patterns that can be documented by an electroencephalogram (EEG), a record of the electrical impulses generated in the brain (see figure 16.1).

During each night a person alternates between nonrapid eye movement (NREM) sleep and rapid eye movement (REM) sleep. The entire cycle of NREM and REM sleep takes about 90 minutes. The average adult sleeps 7.5 hours (five full cycles), with 20 percent of that in REM. By age 70, total sleep time decreases to about 6 hours (four sleep cycles), but the proportion of REM stays at about 20 percent. Sleep efficiency is reduced in elderly persons, with an increased number of awakenings during the night.

In NREM sleep, brain activity, heart rate, respiration, blood pressure, and metabolism (vital signs) slow down and body temperature falls as a deep, restful state is reached. Sleep begins with NREM, during which brain waves gradually lengthen through four distinct stages:

> **Stage 1**—characterized by lighter sleep, a slowing down of brain activity and vital signs, and dreamlike thoughts
>
> **Stage 2**—characterized by slightly deeper sleep and slower vital signs
>
> **Stages 3 and 4 (slow-wave sleep)**—characterized by deep sleep, depressed vital signs, and slow, low-frequency, high-amplitude brain activity known as delta waves

Slow-wave sleep usually terminates with the sleeper's changing position. The brain waves now reverse their course as the sleeper heads for the active REM stage. The central nervous system puts on a display of physiology so intense that Dr. Frederick Snyder of the National Institute of Mental Health terms it "a third stage of earthly existence," distinct from slow-wave sleep and wakefulness.

In REM sleep, the eyes dart about under closed eyelids, and vivid dreams transpire that can often be remembered. The even breathing of NREM gives way to halting uncertainty, and the heart rhythm speeds or

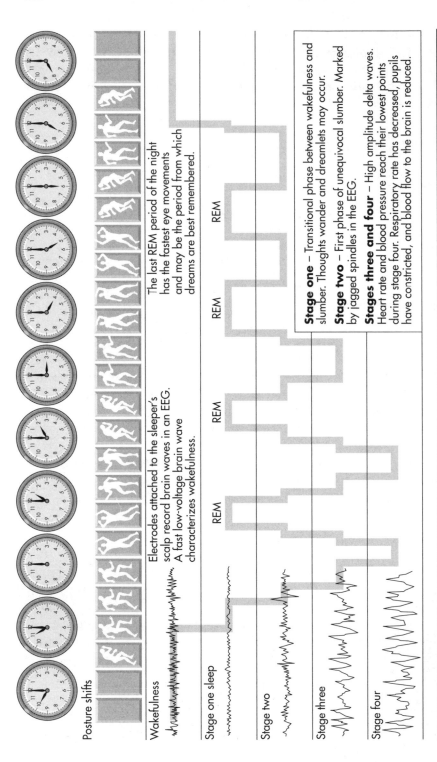

Posture shifts

Wakefulness

Electrodes attached to the sleeper's scalp record brain waves in an EEG. A fast low-voltage brain wave characterizes wakefulness.

Stage one sleep

Stage two

Stage three

Stage four

REM

The last REM period of the night has the fastest eye movements and may be the period from which dreams are best remembered.

**Stage one** – Transitional phase between wakefulness and slumber. Thoughts wander and dreamlets may occur.

**Stage two** – First phase of unequivocal slumber. Marked by jagged spindles in the EEG.

**Stages three and four** – High amplitude delta waves. Heart rate and blood pressure reach their lowest points during stage four. Respiratory rate has decreased, pupils have constricted, and blood flow to the brain is reduced.

**FIGURE 16.1**  A night's sleep consists of four or five cycles, each of which progresses through multiple stages. Adapted, by permission, from "An exercise in sleep." National Geographic, December 1987, 787-789.

slows unaccountably. The brain is highly active during REM sleep, and overall brain metabolism may be increased above the level experienced when awake.

# BETTER SLEEP

Getting a good night's sleep has proven to be a difficult goal for many people in this modern era. Although Solomon once noted that "a lazy man sleeps soundly" (Proverbs 19:15), this option is avoided by most stressed-out, turn-of-the-century men and women.

The Better Sleep Council has published several guidelines for better sleep. "The best time to get a head start on a good night's rest," urges the Better Sleep Council, "is long before you get into bed." Here are eight guidelines for better sleep:

• **Keep regular hours:** According to the Better Sleep Council, sleeping late one morning and rising early the next can lead to a "home-bound version of jet lag." To keep the body's biological clock in order, a regular schedule is "the best way to ensure perfect nights."

• **Cut down on stimulants:** Caffeine from any source (coffee, soft drinks, medications) when taken within six to eight hours of bedtime can make it harder to sleep, diminish deep sleep, and increase nighttime awakenings.

• **Sleep on a good bed:** One is less likely to get deep, solid, restful sleep on a bed that's too small, too soft, too hard, or too old.

• **Don't smoke:** Nicotine is an even stronger stimulant than caffeine. Heavy smokers take longer to fall asleep, awaken more often, and spend less time in REM and deep NREM sleep.

• **Drink only in moderation:** Alcohol late in the evening can suppress REM and deep NREM sleep and accelerate shifts between sleep stages.

• **Set aside a worry or planning time early in the evening:** Sleep is better when anxieties, worries, and possible solutions are dealt with before bedtime.

• **Don't go to bed stuffed or starved:** A big meal late at night forces the digestive system to work overtime, leading to tossing and turning through the night. Going to bed hungry also interferes with sleep.

• **Exercise regularly:** According to the Better Sleep Council, "Exercise enhances sleep by burning off the tensions that accumulate during the day, allowing both body and mind to unwind. While the fit seem to sleep better and deeper . . . you don't have to push to utter exhaustion.

A 20 to 30 minute walk, jog, swim or bicycle ride at least three days a week . . . should be your goal. But don't wait too late in the day to exercise. In the evening, you should be concentrating on winding down rather than working up a sweat. . . . The ideal exercise time is late afternoon or early evening, when your workout can help you shift gears from daytime pressures to evening pleasures."

## EXERCISE-HEALTH CONNECTION

These statements by the Better Sleep Council on the value of exercise in improving the quality and quantity of sleep are based on relatively few well-designed studies. There is considerable debate on the value of exercise in improving sleep, due in large part to the difficulty researchers have in measuring sleep quality.

---

### Does exercise make people sleep better?

In general, those who exercise regularly appear to fall asleep faster and sleep deeper and longer than those who avoid exercise.

---

Compared to those who avoid exercise, physically fit people claim that they fall asleep more rapidly, sleep better, and feel less tired during the day. Scientists have confirmed that people who exercise regularly and intensely do indeed spend more time in slow-wave sleep (a measure of sleep quality) than the inactive. Australian sleep expert, Dr. John Trinder, compared the total amount of time spent in slow-wave sleep between very fit runners (training an average of 45 miles a week) and sedentary controls. The runners spent 18 percent more time in slow-wave sleep than the controls. Dr. Glenn Brassington of San Jose State University compared sleep quality in sedentary and physically active elderly men and women. The exercise group had greater sleep quality in the form of longer sleep duration, shorter time to fall asleep, and better alertness throughout the day. Researchers led by Dr. Sheila Taylor of South Africa have shown that when swimmers increase their levels of training, an increased proportion of sleep time was spent in slow-wave sleep.

Some sleep researchers feel that slow-wave sleep helps restore and revitalize people for the next day. When people initiate and maintain vigorous exercise programs, it would make sense that during sleep they would have to increase the amount of slow-wave sleep to compensate.

In other words, if there is an increase in energy expenditure through exercise, more restoration time in the form of more sleep overall, especially at the deepest level, is required.

Most studies agree with this "theory of restoration." Dr. Karla Kubitz of Kansas State University conducted a comprehensive review of the literature on the effects of exercise on sleep quality and concluded that "individuals who exercise not only fall asleep faster, but also sleep somewhat longer and deeper than individuals who avoid exercise."

An exercise bout has the greatest positive impact on sleep quality for those who are elderly or of low fitness. In other words, those who need it the most gain the greatest sleep benefit from exercise.

The longer the duration of the exercise bout, the better the sleep quality that night, except in the case of unusually severe and prolonged exercise like ultramarathon running races, which can actually disrupt sleep. For example, Dr. Colin Shapiro of Scotland showed that wakefulness in runners was increased on the night following a 92-kilometer race.

There is some evidence that high-intensity exercise leading to sweating has a better effect on sleep quality than does low-intensity exercise. However, researchers do caution that exercising and sweating close to bedtime can have an adverse effect on sleep quality for both fit and sedentary subjects. This is why the Better Sleep Council recommends avoiding heavy exercise late in the day. During slow-wave sleep, the body temperature falls. If physical activities that raise body temperature and cause sweating are conducted too close to bedtime, sleep quality is disturbed because the body and brain are not able to reach the cooler temperatures needed for deep sleep.

Most of the studies on exercise and sleep quality have compared fit and unfit individuals or have analyzed the effect of one exercise bout on that night's sleep. There have been very few exercise training studies to determine whether initiating and maintaining an exercise program improves sleep quality. In one study of new army recruits conducted by Dr. Shapiro, 18 weeks of basic training was found to improve sleep quality by several measures. Most of the sleep quality improvements occurred within the first 9 weeks of training when the recruits were adapting to the increased exercise.

Dr. Abby King from Stanford University assigned physically inactive older adults to exercise or nonexercise groups for 16 weeks. Subjects in the exercise group engaged in low-impact aerobics and brisk walking for 30 to 40 minutes, four days per week. Exercise training led to improved sleep quality, longer sleep, and a shorter time to fall asleep. Dr. King concluded that older adults who often complain of sleep problems "can benefit from initiating a regular moderate-intensity endurance exercise program."

---

### *Does sleep loss impair the ability to exercise?*

Exercise capability is affected little by sleep deprivation, but work performance often decreases due to negative mood states and lack of motivation.

---

It is well documented that lack of sleep negatively affects mood, vigilance, and ability to accomplish complex mental tasks. With regard to the body, most studies have shown that sleep loss of 4 and up to 60 hours does not significantly impair the capability to exercise. However, sleep-deprived subjects still report that the exercise feels harder to accomplish than normal. In other words, the body is able but the mind is unwilling. As summarized by sleep expert Dr. Helen Driver of South Africa, "Following sleep loss of one or two nights, physical performance does not appear to be significantly impaired, provided that participants are sufficiently motivated."

A group of researchers from Canada studied the effects of two days of sleep deprivation on 33 male volunteers. Although the lack of sleep

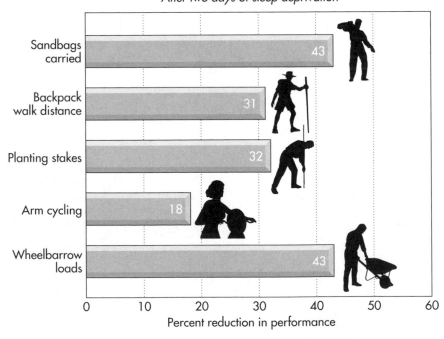

**Decrease in Work/Exercise Performance**
*After two days of sleep deprivation*

FIGURE 16.2    Performance was significantly reduced after two days of sleep deprivation.

had no effect on muscle-power tests, work performance decreased significantly (see figure 16.2). The subjects had a difficult time motivating themselves to do such things as carrying sandbags, walking briskly for 30 minutes, or carrying loads with a wheelbarrow. The researchers concluded that "although sleep-deprived individuals may have the physiological capacity to do the work, the interference of mood, perception of effort or even the repetitive nature of the tasks decreases the ability of individuals to maintain a constant level of work output."

# REFERENCES

Better Sleep Council. (1990). *The sleep better, live better guide.* Washington, DC: Better Sleep Council.

Brassington, G.S., & Hicks, R.A. (1995). Aerobic exercise and self-reported sleep quality in elderly individuals. *Journal of Aging and Physical Activity, 3,* 120-134.

Dement, W.C., & Mitler, M.M. (1993). It's time to wake up to the importance of sleep disorders. *Journal of the American Medical Association, 269,* 1548-1550.

Driver, H.S., & Taylor, S.R. (1996). Sleep disturbances and exercise. *Sports Medicine, 21,* 1-6.

King, A.C., Oman, R.F., Brassington, G.S., Bliwise, D.L., & Haskell, W.L. (1997). Moderate-intensity exercise and self-rated quality of sleep in older adults. *Journal of the American Medical Association, 277,* 32-37.

Kubitz, K.A., Landers, D.M., Petruzzello, S.J., & Han, M. (1996). The effects of acute and chronic exercise on sleep: A meta-analytic review. *Sports Medicine, 21,* 277-291.

Mougin, F., Bourdin, H., Simon-Rigaud, M.L., Didier, J.M., Toubin, G., & Kantelip, J.P. (1996). Effects of a selective sleep deprivation on subsequent anaerobic performance. *International Journal of Sports Medicine, 17,* 115-119.

National Center on Sleep Disorders Research and Office of Prevention, Education, and Control, National Heart, Lung, and Blood Institute, National Institutes of Health. (1994). *Strategy Development Workshop on Sleep Education.* Bethesda, MD: National Institutes of Health.

Nieman, D.C. (1995). *Fitness and sports medicine: A health-related approach.* Menlo Park, CA: Mayfield.

O'Connor, P.J., & Youngstedt, S.D. (1995). Influence of exercise on human sleep. *Exercise and Sport Sciences Reviews, 23,* 105-134.

Rodgers, C.D., Paterson, D.H., Cunningham, D.A., et al. (1995). Sleep deprivation: Effects on work capacity, self-paced walking, contractile properties and perceived exertion. *Sleep, 18,* 30-38.

Shapiro, C.M., Warren, P.M., Trinder, J., et al. (1984). Fitness facilitates sleep. *European Journal of Applied Physiology, 53,* 1-4.

Symons, J.D., VanHelder, T., & Myles, W.S. (1988). Physical performance and physiological responses following 60 hours of sleep deprivation. *Medicine and Science in Sports and Exercise, 20,* 374-380.

Taylor, S.R., Rogers, G.G., and Driver, H.S. (1997). Effects of training volume on sleep, psychological, and physiological profiles of elite female swimmers. *Medicine and Science in Sports and Exercise, 29,* 688-693.

# Chapter 17

# WEIGHT MANAGEMENT

Physical activity might have its most significant effect in preventing, rather than in treating, overweight and obesity.

**Dr. Jack H. Wilmore**

I will have to admit I was surprised when I conducted my first study on the effects of walking on weight loss. After 15 weeks of brisk walking for 45 minutes, five days a week, my overweight female subjects did not lose one pound. How could this be, I asked myself. Since then, I have conducted several other studies, trying to discover the truth about the value of exercise in weight loss. Later in this chapter, I will reveal my findings, which may disappoint and surprise you as much as they first did me.

## Prevalence

Many Americans are preoccupied with weight loss, spending over $30 billion a year in their attempts to become thinner. Using information from four federal surveys, experts convened by the National Institutes of Health have estimated that between 33 and 40 percent of adult women and 20 to 24 percent of men at any given moment are trying to lose weight. Even among high school students, 44 percent of females and 15 percent of males report they are trying to lose weight.

Some have called this the "era of caloric anxiety" in that we have thin standards of beauty but fat ways of living. Despite a nationwide obsession with ideal body weight, government studies over the past 40 years have shown that Americans are losing the war. Obesity, defined as weighing 20 percent more than recommended for a given body height (e.g., 156 pounds instead of 130 pounds for a five-foot, six-inch woman), now afflicts 58 million adults, with the highest rates found among the poor and minority groups.

About one in three American adults is now classified as obese, while about two-thirds weigh more than they should. Among adolescents, one in five is rated as overweight, up substantially from the 1960s.

The federal government's Year 2000 goal is to reduce the prevalence of obesity among adults to no more than 20 percent, but trends are in the opposite direction. Data collected since the 1960s show significant increases in obesity prevalence for all segments of the American society. Several international comparisons have shown that Americans are among the heaviest people in the world.

## Health Hazards

There are many health hazards associated with obesity. Many health experts now feel that obesity constitutes one of the more important medical and public health problems of our era. Researchers have advised that people enjoying the best health are those weighing 15 to 20 percent less than the average American (who tends to be too heavy).

At least eight major health problems are associated with obesity.

- **A psychological burden:** Because of strong pressures from society to be thin, obese people often suffer feelings of guilt, depression, anxiety, and low self-esteem.
- **Increased osteoarthritis:** Overweight persons are at high risk of osteoarthritis in the knees and hips.
- **Increased high blood pressure:** High blood pressure is much more common among the overweight, and the risk climbs strongly with increase in body weight.
- **Increased levels of cholesterol and other blood fats:** Overweight individuals are more likely than normal-weight persons to have high blood cholesterol and triglycerides, as well as lower high-density lipoprotein cholesterol.
- **Increased diabetes:** The prevalence of diabetes is about three times higher among persons who are obese.
- **Increased heart disease:** Not only do people who are obese have more of the risk factors for heart disease, they also die from it at a much higher rate.
- **Increased cancer:** Men and women who are obese have higher cancer death rates for most of the major cancers than do the people who are not obese.
- **Increased early death:** Many researchers have shown that death rates from all causes are higher among people who are obese, while

lean men and women have the lowest death rates. In simple terms, obese people die earlier than those who are lean.

# Theories of Obesity

Explaining why so many Americans weigh more than they should has been a source of confusion to researchers and the public alike. Most obesity experts feel that three factors are most responsible:

• **Genetic and parental influences:** Genetic factors may explain up to 25 percent of the difference in fatness between people. Studies have shown that even when reared apart as infants and children, identical twins by middle age are much closer in body weight than are fraternal twins or siblings. A study of adults who had been adopted before the age of one year revealed that even though they had been brought up by their nonbiological parents, their body weights were still very similar to those of their biological parents. However, in one large study of 6,000 twin pairs in Finland, lifestyle factors were still found to be more important than genetic background in explaining weight gain over a six-year period. Taken together, these studies show that some people are more prone to obesity than others because of genetic factors, and that such persons will have to be unusually careful in their lifestyle habits to counteract these influences.

• **High-calorie, high-fat diets:** There is good reason to believe that the abundance of tasty, calorically rich foods, especially those high in fats, is a major factor explaining the widespread problem of obesity in Western societies. A consistent finding among many researchers is that when the dietary intake of fat is high, most people tend to gain weight rather easily and quickly. When the intake of dietary fats is low, and most calories are in the form of carbohydrate, desirable body weight is more readily achieved.

• **Insufficient energy expenditure:** People burn calories in three ways. As shown in figure 17.1, about two-thirds of the daily energy expenditure is from the resting metabolism, 23 percent is from physical activity, and 10 percent is from food digestion and utilization.

The resting metabolic rate (RMR) is defined as the energy expended by the body to maintain life and normal body functions. The RMR is closely tied to body size, with large people having the highest amplitude. In other words, people who are obese have higher RMRs than those who are lean because of their greater body mass. Some researchers have determined that a low RMR among normal-weight people is a risk factor for future obesity, but this has not been a consistent finding. One

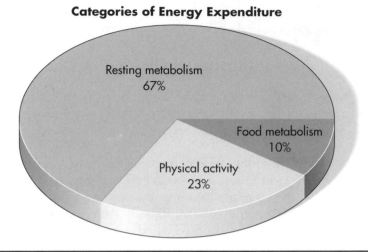

**Categories of Energy Expenditure**

FIGURE 17.1   Daily energy expenditure for the average person.

thing that researchers do agree on is that individuals who are obese tend to exercise less than those who are lean.

## Treatment of Obesity

Losing weight and then keeping it off has proven to be one of the most difficult of all health challenges. According to health professionals who treat obesity, many overweight people will not stay in treatment. Of those who do, most will not achieve ideal body weight, and of those who lose weight, most will regain it.

For most weight loss methods, there are few scientific studies evaluating their effectiveness and safety. Studies that are available indicate that people can be quite successful losing weight in the short term, but that after completing the program or weight loss scheme they tend to quickly regain the weight.

For example, in a four-year study of 152 men and women who had participated in a 15-week weight loss program including diet, exercise, and behavior modification, less than 3 percent of subjects were able to maintain posttreatment weights throughout the four years of follow-up. In another study, only 5 percent of subjects maintained all of their weight loss after five years, while 18 percent maintained a loss greater than 11 pounds.

According to experts, obesity has typically been treated as if it is an acute illness like the flu, when it is more appropriately viewed as a chronic condition (like heart disease or diabetes). Since the ultimate goal of a weight-reduction program is to lose weight and maintain the loss, a nutritionally balanced, low-energy diet that is applicable to the patient's lifestyle is most appropriate. A comprehensive weight-reduction program that incorporates diet, exercise, and behavior modification is more likely to lead to long-term weight control.

For most individuals who are obese, a weight loss of about 1 percent total body weight per week is optimal. For example, a woman who weighs 150 pounds but wants to weigh 130 pounds should lose no more than an average of 1 to 1.5 pounds a week. Since each pound of body fat represents about 3,500 calories, this would require expending 500 to 750 calories more than the amount taken in through the diet. This could be accomplished by increasing energy expenditure through physical activity by 200 to 300 calories a day and reducing dietary fat intake by 300 to 450 calories. Each tablespoon of fat represents about 100 calories, so an emphasis on low-fat dairy products and lean meats, and a low intake of visible fats (oils, butter, margarine, salad dressings, sour cream, etc.), would be the easiest way to reduce caloric intake without reducing the volume of food eaten.

According to most weight-management experts, treatment for obesity should involve three elements:

- **Diet:** The caloric intake should be reduced, preferably by reducing the fat content of the diet while increasing intake of carbohydrates and dietary fiber (e.g., whole grains, fruits, and vegetables).

- **Exercise:** Energy expenditure should be increased at least 200 to 400 calories per day through an increase in all forms of physical activity.

- **Behavior modification:** Several techniques should be employed, including:

  *-Self-monitoring:* People can keep diet diaries, emphasizing recording of food amounts consumed and circumstances surrounding the eating episode.

  *-Control of the events that precede eating:* People can identify and control the circumstances that elicit eating and overeating (e.g., avoiding reading or watching television while eating, or staying away from food when depressed or stressed).

  *-Development of techniques to control the act of eating:* Typical behavioral modification techniques are used such as slowing down the eating process, putting the fork down between bites, keeping the serving sizes moderate, eating only at defined times and places, and the like.

*-Reinforcement through use of rewards:* A system of formal rewards facilitates progress. For example, close friends could arrange for a special gift, trip, or award for meeting established goals.

## EXERCISE-HEALTH CONNECTION

Exercise can influence body weight from three different angles: prevention of weight gain, treatment of obesity, and maintenance of desirable body weight following weight loss. In this chapter, each approach will be discussed, starting with prevention.

---

### Can regular exercise help prevent weight gain during adulthood?

Yes. Most studies of large population groups have determined that lean people are more active than obese individuals and that regular exercise reduces the odds of gaining weight with age.

---

Most studies have shown that obese children and adults are less active than normal-weight people. Obese men, for example, have been found to walk about 3.7 miles during the normal course of their day as compared to 6 miles for normal-weight men. Obese people tend to stay in bed longer and spend 15 to 20 percent less time on their feet; and when given the choice of an escalator or stairs, they are more likely than the lean to take the escalator. Several investigations have shown that the risk of obesity among adolescents and adults rises with the number of hours viewing television. Researchers surmise that the TV viewing prompts extra snacking and takes the place of more active pursuits.

In general, many studies indicate that physical activity decreases in direct relationship to the degree of obesity. However, as researchers readily admit, it has been difficult to determine whether the inactivity causes obesity or whether the obesity leads to the inactivity. It's probably both, with a vicious cycle setting in. Long-term inactivity appears to promote gain in body weight, and then physical activity becomes more onerous.

Figure 17.2 shows the results of one large study conducted by the Centers for Disease Control and Prevention (CDC). For both men and women, those reporting regular and intense physical activity had a much lower prevalence of obesity than their inactive counterparts. However, as the CDC researchers were quick to point out, "It is important to consider that these are cross-sectional data, and therefore causality between physical activity and weight cannot be inferred directly.

### Prevalence of Overweight by Physical Activity Pattern
CDC BRFSS, 6,125 men, 12,557 women

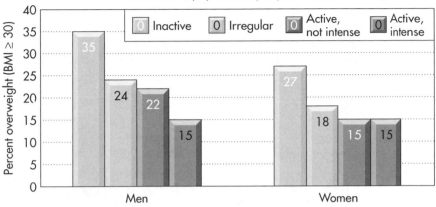

FIGURE 17.2  Overweight prevalence is highest among physically inactive men and women.

Based on data from DiPietro L, et al, 1993.

Indeed, physical activity patterns and choices may be determined by weight, just as weight may be influenced by physical activity."

There is some indication that long-term physical activity is related to a lower risk of gaining weight. Researchers from the American Cancer Institute followed over 79,000 people for 10 years and found that those engaging in vigorous exercise one to three hours a week, or walking for more than four hours a week, were better able to ward off weight gain than their more sedentary counterparts.

When a group of over 9,000 men and women were followed for 10 years, major weight gain was much more likely among people with low versus high amounts of physical activity. In this study, however, researchers could not determine whether the exercise countered the weight gain or whether regular physical activity served as a marker of people who were unusually disciplined and careful in all aspects of their lifestyle, including diet. In other words, people who are motivated enough to exercise faithfully may also be unusually vigilant in their dietary habits, enough to keep their weight under good control. Once again, the answer may be both—regular exercise counters weight gain and distinguishes those who display proper dietary restraint.

It should be underscored that most adult Americans gain weight slowly, about one pound a year on average according to most estimates. At the same time, muscle mass is slowly lost while body fat increases. This slow change in the quality and quantity of body weight is very easily countered by regular exercise if the diet is also kept under good control.

Dr. Jack Wilmore of the University of Texas in Austin, a leading expert in exercise and obesity, feels that although more research is needed, what is known about exercise and prevention of weight gain is very impressive. "Increasing amounts of physical activity or maintaining high levels of physical activity for purposes of weight control might be most important in preventing the increases in weight known to occur with aging, from the early 20s through the late 60s," summarizes Dr. Wilmore.

---

### If I exercise while I diet, will I lose weight faster?

If the exercise is at moderate levels, the actual amount of energy expended tends to be lower than expected, and has a rather small impact on weight loss during the two to six months of the reducing diet.

---

Although it is widely accepted that physical activity is a powerful tool in promoting weight loss during a two- to four-month weight loss program, the best-designed research studies have failed to strongly support this belief. In fact, most researchers in this area now regard exercise as a relatively weak weapon in accelerating weight loss during dieting, with control of caloric intake representing the real power behind weight loss efforts.

There are several misconceptions regarding the role of exercise in weight loss:

- That exercise accelerates weight loss significantly when combined with a reducing diet
- That exercise causes the RMR to stay elevated for a long time after the bout, burning extra calories
- That it counters the diet-induced decrease in RMR
- That it counters the diet-induced decrease in fat-free mass

Some people who are obese have been led to believe that if they start brisk walking two to three miles a day, significant amounts of body weight will be lost quickly. Most research is not supportive of this idea, even when the exercise program lasts several months.

For example, in a carefully conducted one-year study of 350 men and women at Stanford University, three or five 30- to 40-minute exercise sessions per week had no significant effect on body weight despite a 5 to 8 percent improvement in aerobic fitness. In other words, the exercise made the subjects fitter but did not make them leaner.

A team of researchers from Loughborough University in England had women walk 2.5 hours a week for a whole year and were unable to measure any decrease in body fat, even though the women did not appear to change their diets. The researchers concluded that the walkers may have rested more throughout the day after their walk, erasing the effects of the walking session.

Many other studies have come to the same conclusion, that when young and old alike exercise moderately (e.g., walking for 30 to 45 minutes, several times a week), this amount of exercise ends up being an insufficient stimulus to reduce body weight appreciably when there are no formal attempts to alter the diet.

It has been argued that when people begin exercising, they may start eating more, canceling out the extra calories burned from the exercise. Or perhaps they may alter other areas of their lifestyle (e.g., relax more than normal during the rest of the day after exercise), diluting the effect of added exercise. In other words, it is the tendency of many people to "reward" themselves for exercising by eating or resting more than normal.

For these reasons, many researchers have tested the effects of exercise under controlled dietary conditions, in which all subjects are fed the same amount of food while some exercise and others remain sedentary. Even under these conditions, moderate amounts of exercise have been found to add little to the weight loss, at least in the short term (two to six months).

Dr. Joseph Donnelly of Kearney State College in Nebraska put 69 obese females on a 520-calorie liquid-formula diet for three months and tested the effects of four hours per week of exercise on weight loss, lean body weight, and metabolism. Subjects were randomized into one of four groups: diet only, diet plus aerobic training, diet plus weight training, and diet plus aerobic and weight training. Aerobic training consisted of four sessions a week, with duration increasing from 20 minutes up to 60 minutes per session by the end of the study, at 70 percent intensity. The weight trainers exercised four times a week, engaging in two to three sets, six to eight repetitions of several exercises at 70 to 80 percent of maximum.

Whether subjects exercised or not, all lost an average of 45 to 50 pounds, with three-fourths of the weight loss measured as fat and one-fourth as lean body weight. According to Dr. Donnelly, "This study did not identify any advantage of using exercise in combination with a diet over a diet alone with respect to metabolism, body-weight loss, or the type of weight lost." (See figure 17.3.)

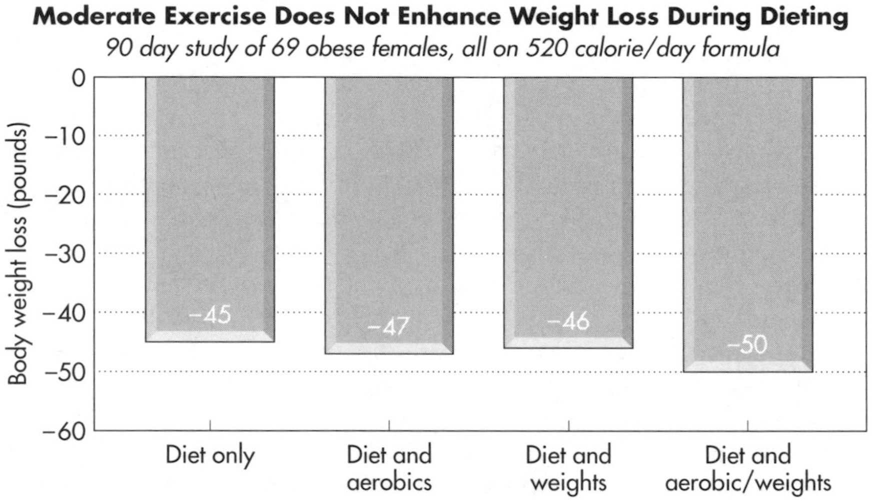

**Moderate Exercise Does Not Enhance Weight Loss During Dieting**

*90 day study of 69 obese females, all on 520 calorie/day formula*

FIGURE 17.3   During 90 days of dieting, moderate exercise did not significantly accelerate weight loss.

Based on data from Donnelly, J.E. et al., 1991.

These and other studies demonstrate that when moderate amounts of aerobic exercise (two to seven hours per week) are combined with a reducing diet, weight loss is not accelerated much beyond a few extra pounds at best. It appears that if aerobic exercise is to have a major effect on weight loss, daily exercise sessions need to be unusually long in duration (more than one hour) and high in intensity—something that most overweight people cannot do (or do not wish to do). Although this may seem somewhat surprising, when the numbers are added up the actual number of calories expended during moderate exercise is rather modest—and much less than most people believe.

The net energy cost of exercise equals the calories expended during the exercise session minus the calories expended for the RMR and other activities that would have occupied the individual had he or she not been formally exercising. For example, the net energy cost of a three-mile, 45-minute walk for a 154-pound woman is only about 130 to 140 calories. The math is as follows:

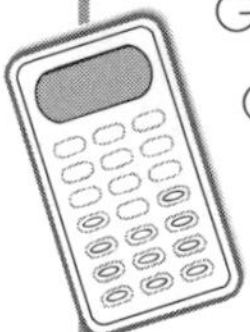

| | |
|---|---|
| Gross number of calories burned during 45-minute walk: | 215 calories |
| Calories burned by the resting metabolism during walk: | −50 calories |
| Calories typically burned if not walking for 45 minutes: | −30 calories |
| Net energy expenditure: | 135 calories |

In other words, if the woman were not walking for 45 minutes, she would still be burning calories through her resting metabolism and incidental activities. Thus the net energy expenditure is only about 135 calories for a 45-minute brisk walk.

Since one pound of human fat contains approximately 3,500 calories, if all else stayed exactly the same it would take nearly one month of daily brisk walking (three miles each session) to lose one pound of fat. Many who are obese find walking two to three miles a day to be the most they can handle without injury, yet much more than this is necessary if significant weight loss is to be achieved.

It should be noted that two to three miles of walking a day should lead to one pound of body weight loss per month *if* all else stayed the same. As indicated earlier in this section, however, many people tend to eat more or make other adjustments in their daily routine, negating the extra calories burned.

As emphasized by University of Vermont obesity researchers, "The types and intensities of exercise that carry a high energy expenditure for a single bout are basically confined to those that can be undertaken by elite athletes or subjects with an excellent level of physical fitness. On a clinical basis, and especially for the obese patient, it would be unrealistic (even dangerous) to expect such a level of exercise performance."

The practical advice to be derived from these studies is that exercise must not be seen as the one and only major weapon in the treatment of obesity. Instead, improvements in the quality and quantity of the diet should take the lead, with exercise relegated to an important supporting role.

At the 1992 National Institutes of Health Technology Assessment Conference Panel on Methods for Voluntary Weight Loss and Control, it was concluded: "Weight loss that can be achieved by exercise programs alone is more limited than that which can be obtained by caloric restriction. However, exercise has beneficial effects independent of weight loss . . . and can be an important adjunct to other strategies."

---

### Will exercise cause my body to burn calories for a long time after an exercise session?

There is a slight increase in RMR for a short time after moderate exercise. The actual amount of extra energy expended (10 to 30 calories) is too small to have a meaningful effect on body weight.

---

Another common misconception is that aerobic exercise causes the RMR to stay elevated for a long time after the bout, burning extra calories. In general, most researchers have found that the energy expended after aerobic exercise is small unless the amount of high-intensity exercise has been great.

For example, jogging (12 minutes per mile), walking, or cycling at moderate intensities for about one-half hour causes the RMR to stay elevated for 20 to 30 minutes, burning 10 to 12 extra calories. When the intensity is increased to higher levels, RMR is increased for about 35 to 45 minutes, with 15 to 30 extra calories expended. For the obese individual who takes a 20- to 30-minute walk, about 10 extra calories at most will be burned during recovery, hardly enough to be meaningful when balanced against other factors.

Even when the exercise is at athletic levels (long duration, high intensity), the number of calories expended afterward through elevation of the RMR is rather low (about 100 to 200 calories).

---

### I know that my resting metabolism (RMR) gets lower when I diet. Will exercise help my RMR stay higher?

Dieting can cause the resting metabolism to fall 10 to 30 percent, depending on how severe the decrease in energy intake is. Moderate amounts of exercise appear to have little if any effect in countering this decrease.

---

During dieting, the RMR drops substantially, and the size of the decrease is related to the rate of weight loss, averaging 10 to 20 percent for low-calorie diets (400 to 800 calories per day) and up to 20 to 30 percent for long-term fasting. Can exercise during caloric restriction counter this diet-induced decrease in the RMR?

Most studies are not supportive of this idea. For example, in one investigation 12 mildly obese women were put onto 530-calorie diets for 28 days and into an exercise program (three sessions per week, 30 to 45 minutes at a moderate intensity). Resting metabolic rate dropped 16 percent despite the exercise program. In a 90-day study of moderately obese women on a 520 calorie per day diet, neither aerobic or weight training had any effect in countering the 10 percent drop in metabolism caused by the diet. Even on 1,200 to 1,500 calories per day, the RMR will drop slightly (about 5 percent), and exercise has no countering effect.

In another study, half of 13 mildly obese subjects on a four-week low-calorie diet (720 calories per day) exercised 45 to 60 minutes a day moderately. The RMR actually dropped more in the exercise group than in the sedentary group. Exercise during low-calorie diets may actually prompt the body to slow down the RMR to conserve energy.

---

### I don't want to lose muscle weight or water weight when I diet. Will exercise help me avoid that?

Most studies have shown that dieting causes some loss of muscle and water weight (fat-free mass), and that moderate amounts of aerobic and/or weight training are an insufficient stimulus to alter the decrease.

---

During weight loss, the percentage of body weight lost as fat-free mass (FFM or water, muscle, and other nonfat tissues) increases in relation to the severity of the diet. During total fasting, for example, the body weight loss is split about evenly between fat and FFM. During a low-calorie diet (400 to 800 calories per day), about 75 percent of the weight loss is fat and 25 percent is FFM. During a 1,200- to 1,500-calorie diet, about 90 percent of the weight loss is fat and only 10 percent is FFM.

Can exercise counter the diet-induced decrease in FFM (if this is the desire of the overweight individual)? In general, both moderate aerobic and strength-training programs have been found to have little effect. For example, in the 90-day study of overweight women on a 520-calorie diet referred to earlier (see figure 17.3), FFM represented about 22 percent of the 45 to 50 pounds lost, and moderate aerobic and/or weight training had no effect on this proportion.

In another 90-day study of moderately obese females who were on an 800-calorie diet, weight training three times a week did not counter the 25 percent decrease in FFM. In general, it appears that exercise is an insufficient stimulus to alter the diet-induced drop in FFM.

---

### What are the chief benefits of exercise for weight loss?

In general, regular exercise helps to counter many of the obesity-related diseases and health problems. Long-term exercise is a vital factor together with prudent dietary habits to keep body weight under good control and to build physical fitness.

---

If exercise training has relatively little effect during weight loss programs in accelerating weight loss, or in protecting diet-induced decreases in the RMR and FFM, then why should overweight individuals exercise?

The main reason is to improve health. Moderate exercise may be a weak weapon in promoting a great deal of weight loss, but it has much greater power in enhancing health. There are at least five health-related benefits of exercise for obese patients:

- Improved cardiorespiratory endurance ($\dot{V}O_2max$)
- Improved blood lipid profile, in particular decreased triglycerides and increased high-density lipoprotein cholesterol, with weight loss more responsible for decreases in total cholesterol and low-density lipoprotein cholesterol
- Improved psychological state, especially increased general well-being and vigor and decreased anxiety and depression
- Decreased risk of obesity-related diseases (e.g., diabetes, heart disease, cancer, hypertension)
- Enhanced long-term maintenance of weight loss

According to the American Health Foundation's Expert Panel on Healthy Weight, "Because physically active people have a lower risk of chronic diseases associated with overweight, regular physical activity should be advocated for the prevention of weight gain and the maintenance of a stable weight. At least 30 minutes of moderate physical activity per day should be incorporated into the goals for a healthier lifestyle."

So in summary, moderate aerobic exercise during weight reduction helps to improve the health and fitness status of the individual, while the real power behind weight loss comes from a reduction in the number of calories (in particular, the dietary fat) consumed. However, as will be emphasized in the next section, regular exercise has surfaced as one of the best ways to improve long-term maintenance of the weight loss.

---

### I've recently lost weight. How important is exercise in keeping the weight off?

Regular exercise has emerged as one of the best predictors of those who are able to maintain weight loss over the long term.

---

Obesity experts have urged that more vigorous efforts be put forth to help overweight people maintain weight loss following programs. The experts recommend that patients participate in at least a 6- to 12-month program of weight loss maintenance immediately after losing weight (no matter what the method), and that they be prepared to reenter therapy whenever they show a gain of 10 pounds or more that they cannot reverse on their own.

Several studies have analyzed factors that predict long-term maintenance of weight loss after participation in a weight loss program. In one study of 509 obese subjects, predictors of success after two years were feeling in control of eating habits, success during actual treatment, frequency of weight measurement, and increase in physical activity. Another study of 118 obese patients who were followed for more than three years showed that weight loss was maintained best in those who reported eating fewer high-fat foods, using the behavioral techniques taught in the program, and exercising more.

Several other studies have found that one of the best markers for long-term success in weight loss is participation in regular exercise. Investigators showed that 90 percent of women who had lost weight and maintained their losses for more than two years reported engaging in regular exercise as compared with only 34 percent of the women who had regained their weight losses.

Dr. Francine Grodstein of Harvard University surveyed 192 obese individuals who had participated in a weight loss program three years previously. The average person had lost 48 pounds; but only 12 percent had maintained three-fourths of their weight loss in the three years after leaving the diet program, while 40 percent had gained back more than they had lost. Of all factors measured, the frequency of exercise ended up being the strongest predictor of weight loss maintenance, while television viewing best predicted a gain in weight.

Researchers at the University of Pittsburgh and University of Colorado have formed a national registry of people who have lost more than 30 pounds and kept it off for more than a year. Several hundred people are now in this registry, and several interesting findings have emerged:

- 94 percent of successful losers increased their physical activity level to accomplish their weight loss, with walking the most common activity reported.
- 92 percent report that they are continuing to exercise to maintain weight loss.
- 98 percent decreased their food intake in some way.
- 57 percent received professional help from physicians, registered dietitians, Weight Watchers, and others.

"We have to debunk the myth that there are no successful losers," urges Dr. Rena Wing, who heads up the registry. "There's no magic to why people lose and keep it off. They just keep exercising and watching what they eat."

According to Dr. John Foreyt of Baylor College of Medicine in Houston, "Exercise is one of the most reliable predictors of success in weight loss maintenance." In other words, even though exercise does not help one lose large amounts of body weight quickly, if the goal is avoiding weight regain, regular exercise may be the key.

# REFERENCES

Ching, P.L.Y.H., Willett, W.C., Rimm, E.B., Colditz, G.A., Gortmaker, S.L., & Stampfer, M.J. (1996). Activity level and risk of overweight in male health professionals. *American Journal of Public Health, 86,* 25-30.

DiPietro, L. (1995). Physical activity, body weight, and adiposity: An epidemiologic perspective. *Exercise and Sport Sciences Reviews, 23,* 275-303.

DiPietro, L., Williamson, D.F., Caspersen, C.J., & Eaker, E. (1993). The descriptive epidemiology of selected physical activities and body weight among adults trying to lose weight: The Behavioral Risk Factor Surveillance System Survey, 1989. *International Journal of Obesity, 17,* 69-76.

Donnelly, J.E., Pronk, N.P., & Jacobsen, D.J. (1991). Effects of a very-low-calorie diet and physical training regimens on body composition and resting metabolic rate in obese females. *American Journal of Clinical Nutrition, 54,* 56-61.

Grodstein, F., Levine, R., Troy, L., Spencer, T., Colditz, G.A., & Stampfer, M.J. (1996). Three-year follow-up of participants in a commercial weight loss program. *Archives of Internal Medicine, 156,* 1302-1306.

Korkeila, M., Kaprio, J., Rissanen, A., & Koskenvuo, M. (1995). Consistency and change of body mass index and weight. A study on 5967 adult Finnish twin pairs. *International Journal of Obesity, 19,* 310-317.

Manson, J.E., Willett, W.C., Stampfer, M.J., et al. (1995). Body weight and mortality among women. *New England Journal of Medicine, 333,* 677-685.

Meisler, J.G., & St. Jeor, S. (1996). Summary and recommendations from the American Health Foundation's Expert Panel on Healthy Weight. *American Journal of Clinical Nutrition, 63* (Suppl.), 474S-477S.

Nieman, D.C. (1995). *Fitness and sports medicine: A health-related approach.* Mountain Park, CA: Mayfield.

Willett, W.C., Manson, J.E., Stampfer, M.J., et al. (1995). Weight, weight change, and coronary heart disease in women. *Journal of the American Medical Association, 273,* 461-465.

Williams, M.J., Hunter, G.R., Kekes-Szabo, T., Snyder, S., & Treuth, M.S. (1997). Regional fat distribution in women and risk of cardiovascular disease. *American Journal of Clinical Nutrition, 65*, 855-860.

Wilmore, J.H. (1996). Increasing physical activity: Alterations in body mass and composition. *American Journal of Clinical Nutrition, 63* (Suppl.), 456S-460S.

# Chapter 18

# STRESS MANAGEMENT

A turn or two I'll walk, to still my beating mind.

Shakespeare, *Cymbeline*, Act III

Dr. Hans Selye, who earlier in this century pioneered the concept of stress, conducted an interesting experiment to demonstrate the remarkable anti-stress benefits of walking. In his experiment, conducted at the University of Montreal where he was a professor, Dr. Selye subjected 10 rats to a month-long program of electric shocks, blinding lights, and loud noises. At the end of the month all 10 of the animals were dead because of the negative impact this stress had on their health.

During the second phase of this experiment, Dr. Selye had 10 rats walk on treadmills until they were in good physical condition, and then subjected them to the same stress program as before. At the end of one month, all 10 of the physically active rats remained alive and reasonably well. Dr. Selye concluded that physical fitness "buffered" the rats against the health-destroying effects of stress.

In this chapter, emphasis will be placed on the benefits of exercise on psychological well-being and mental health. This is considered one of the chief advantages of regular exercise. According to the 1996 Surgeon General's report on physical activity and health, a major conclusion of experts in this area was that "physical activity improves mental health." According to the document's summary, "The literature reported here supports a beneficial effect of physical activity on relieving symptoms of depression and anxiety and on improving mood."

## STRESS PROBLEMS

Improved mental health and management of stress are topics of great interest to modern-day men and women. Mental health is a general term used to refer to the absence of mental disorders and the ability to negotiate successfully the daily challenges and social interactions of life.

Many Americans are falling short. During any one-year period, an estimated 52 million American adults (about 3 in 10) experience some form of mental disorder, imposing a $148 billion cost burden. The National Institute of Mental Health has estimated that the top three mental health problems in the United States are as follows:

| | |
|---|---|
| Anxiety disorders | 23.3 million Americans |
| Depression | 17.6 million |
| Substance abuse disorders | 17.5 million |

According to the U.S. Public Health Service, during any given two-week period about 6 in 10 Americans report experiencing at least a moderate amount of stress, while nearly 1 in 5 experiences "great stress" almost every day. Negative moods such as feeling lonely, restless, bored, or upset are reported by a substantial number of U.S. adults.

## The Stress Response

Stress has been defined as any action or situation (stressor) that places special physical or psychological demands on a person—in other words, anything that unbalances one's equilibrium. Dr. Selye wrote in his 1956 classic, *The Stress of Life,* that "stress is essentially the rate of wear and tear in the body."

There are two types of stress: eustress and distress. Eustress is good stress and appears to motivate and inspire (e.g., falling in love, or exercising moderately). Distress is considered bad stress, and can be acute (quite intense, but then disappears quickly) or chronic (not so intense, but lingers for prolonged periods of time).

Dr. Selye observed that whether a situation was perceived as very good (e.g., getting married) or very bad (e.g., getting divorced), demands were placed upon the body and mind, forcing them to adapt. According to Dr. Selye, the physiological response or arousal was very similar during both good and bad situations, producing a similar physiological response.

Medical research on the effects of stress dates back to the early part of the 1900s when Dr. Walter Cannon of Harvard University first coined the term "fight-or-flight response," now known as the stress response. In this response, the muscles tense and tighten, breathing becomes deep and fast, the heart rate rises and blood vessels constrict, blood pressure rises, the stomach and intestines temporarily halt digestion, perspiration increases, the thyroid gland is stimulated, secretion of saliva slows, blood sugar and fats rise, and sensory perception becomes sharper. These responses are regulated by the nervous system and various hormones, redirecting energy, oxygen, and fuel to allow the body to cope with the physical or emotional stress (see figure 18.1).

In the 1940s and 1950s, Dr. Selye extended Dr. Cannon's work, laying the foundation for today's understanding of stress and its medical consequences. Experimenting with rats while using various physical stressors such as cold temperature or random electrical shock, Dr. Selye discovered that if the stressor was maintained long enough, the body would go through three stages:

- Alarm reaction (essentially the fight-or-flight response)
- Stage of resistance (body functions would return to normal as the body adjusted)
- Stage of exhaustion (alarm reaction symptoms return, leading to disease and death)

Dr. Selye and other stress researchers, however, urged that not all stress is harmful. In fact, it appears that human beings need some degree of stress to stay healthy. While the human body needs some sort of balance (homeostasis or physiological calm), it also requires arousal to ensure that the heart, muscles, lungs, nerves, brain, and other tissues stay in good shape.

# ILL EFFECTS OF HIGH STRESS

Chronic stressors (e.g., economic difficulties, intolerable relationships, bodily pain) are thought to be the real villains and have been associated with a growing list of health and disease problems. Chronic anxiety and depression, an overabundance of life-change events, and repressed feelings of loss, bereavement, emotional distress, and hostility have been linked to increased risk of heart disease, cancer, infection, suppressed immunity, asthma attacks, back pain, chronic fatigue, gastrointestinal distress, headaches, and insomnia.

For example, Dr. John Barefoot studied 740 men and women of Glostrup, Denmark, and found that chronic depression was related to a 70-percent increased risk of heart attack over a 20-year period. In a study of some 1,000 men, followed for 30 years, those who had the highest anger scores on a psychological test taken in their 20s were about three times more likely to have a heart attack and nearly six times more likely to have a stroke during midlife.

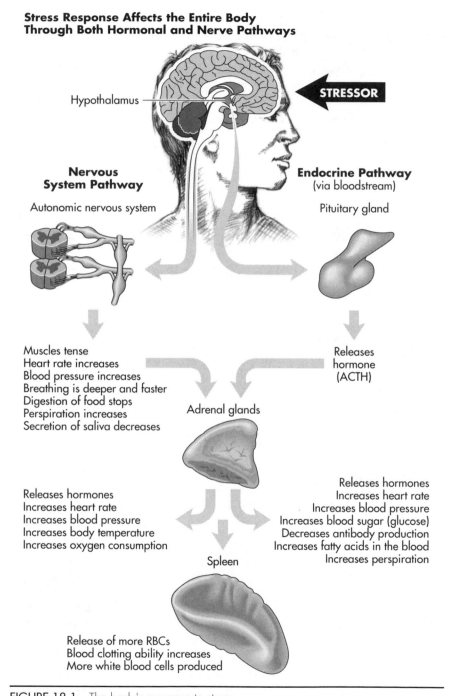

**Stress Response Affects the Entire Body
Through Both Hormonal and Nerve Pathways**

STRESSOR

Hypothalamus

**Nervous
System Pathway**

Autonomic nervous system

**Endocrine Pathway**
(via bloodstream)

Pituitary gland

Muscles tense
Heart rate increases
Blood pressure increases
Breathing is deeper and faster
Digestion of food stops
Perspiration increases
Secretion of saliva decreases

Releases
hormone
(ACTH)

Adrenal glands

Releases hormones
Increases heart rate
Increases blood pressure
Increases body temperature
Increases oxygen consumption

Releases hormones
Increases heart rate
Increases blood pressure
Increases blood sugar (glucose)
Decreases antibody production
Increases fatty acids in the blood
Increases perspiration

Spleen

Release of more RBCs
Blood clotting ability increases
More white blood cells produced

FIGURE 18.1    The body's response to stress.
From *Fitness & Sports Medicine: A Health Related Approach* by David C. Nieman. Copyright © 1995
by Mayfield Publishing Company. Adapted by permission of the publisher.

Swedish researchers asked some 7,000 men how often they had trouble sleeping or felt tense, irritable, or anxious. Over the next 12 years, the men who said they constantly experienced those symptoms were about 70 percent more likely to die of a heart attack or stroke than the other men were. Another Swedish study, involving nearly a million people, linked stressful jobs—jobs that involved high pressure or gave the worker little power to make decisions—with a 60-percent increase in heart attack risk.

Researchers at Carnegie Mellon University injected cold viruses into the noses of some 400 volunteers and reported that the risk of coming down with a cold was directly related to the stress levels of the subjects. Those experiencing the most stress and tension were almost twice as likely to catch cold as those who reported the least. Researchers in Australia found that stressed people had twice as many days with flu and cold symptoms compared to those reporting little stress during a six-month period. Marital disruption has been linked to depressed immunity and physical illness, with separated partners having about 30 percent more acute illnesses and physician visits than those who remain married.

# STRESS MANAGEMENT

Obviously many people need to learn how to manage stress. Stress management revolves around five major principles:

- **Controlling stressors:** Although stressors are omnipresent, they can be modified, reduced in number, avoided, or controlled. Just as in climbing a mountain with a backpack, one can manage stressors by controlling the pace and the load carried.

- **Managing stress reactions:** Marcus Aurelius once noted, "If you are distressed by anything external, the pain is not due to the thing itself, but to your estimate of it. This you have the power to revoke at any time." In other words, the mind can choose a more positive response to any particular stressful event, avoiding the negative health effects of the stress response.

- **Seeking the social support of others:** Seeking others' social support and sharing emotional, social, physical, financial, and other types of comfort and assistance have been related to improved health, while social isolation has been linked to impaired health and increased risk of disease.

- **Finding satisfaction in service to others:** Dr. Albert Schweitzer wrote, "I don't know what your destiny will be. But I do know that the only ones among you who will find true happiness are those who find a place to serve." Dr. Selye added, "My own code is based on the view that to achieve peace of mind and fulfillment through self-expression, most men need a commitment to work in the service of some cause that they can respect."

- **Keeping healthy:** Stressors appear to have less of a negative impact, according to some stress researchers, when the body is healthy from adequate sleep, exercise, relaxation, and a prudent diet.

## EXERCISE-HEALTH CONNECTION

The part of the brain that enables us to exercise, the motor cortex, lies only a few millimeters away from the part of the brain strata that deals with thought and feeling. Might their proximity mean that when exercise stimulates the motor cortex it has a parallel effect on cognition, emotion, and psychological mood state?

Since the beginning of time many have believed in the "cerebral satisfaction" of exercise. The Greeks maintained that exercise made their minds more lucid. Aristotle started his "Peripatetic School" in 335 B.C. The school was so named because of Aristotle's habit of walking up and down (*peripaton*) the paths of the Lyceum in Athens while thinking or lecturing to the students who walked with him. Plato and Socrates had also practiced the art of peripatetics as did later the Roman *Ordo Vagorum* or walking scholars. Centuries later, Oliver Wendell Holmes explained that "in walking the will and the muscles are so accustomed to working together and perform their task with so little expenditure of force that the intellect is left comparatively free."

---

*Do physically active and fit people have better psychological well-being than their sedentary peers?*

Surveys and cross-sectional comparisons of physically active and inactive adults nearly all show that regular exercise is linked to good mental health. However, many factors other than physical activity may contribute to this finding.

---

Many investigators have surveyed physically active and inactive people, comparing measures of psychological well-being, anxiety, depression, and mood state. In the midst of the fitness revolution in the United States, the "Perrier Survey of Fitness in America" conducted by Louis Harris and Associates in 1978 showed that those with a deep commitment to exercise reported feeling more relaxed, less tired, and more disciplined; the exercisers also reported a sense of looking better, greater self-confidence, greater productivity in work, and in general, being more at one with themselves.

The 1988 Campbell's Survey on Well-Being in Canada revealed that physically active people reported less depression and higher levels of positive well-being than their inactive peers. Other surveys have shown that when physically active people are asked why they exercise, the most common response is "to feel better mentally and physically." A survey by *Runner's World* magazine implied that although most people start running to "improve physical fitness," most continue to run to "improve mental fitness" and to "relieve stress." A *Men's Health/CNN* survey conducted in the mid-1990s showed that men say they exercise to stay healthy (78 percent), raise sense of well-being (54 percent), control stress (50 percent), and control weight (47 percent).

Dr. Tom Stephens of Canada directed the evaluation of data from four national surveys in the United States and Canada. People reporting "much exercise" scored highest in psychological well-being in comparison to other groups reporting less exercise. "The inescapable conclusion from these four national studies," summarized Dr. Stephens, "is that physical activity is positively associated with good mental health, especially positive mood, general well-being, and less anxiety and depression." This relationship was found to be stronger for the older age group (40-plus years of age) than for the younger, and for women than for men.

In one cross-sectional study of elderly women, psychological well-being scores were found to be significantly better among highly conditioned versus sedentary elderly women (average age, 73 years). The highly conditioned women had been exercising for an average of 11 years, trained about 1.5 hours a day, and were active in state and national senior games competitions (see figure 18.2).

The problem with these kinds of studies, however, is that physically active people are often quite different from their inactive peers in many other lifestyle and demographic factors including diet, body weight, sleep habits, education, income, and genetic endowment. These other factors make it difficult to measure the independent role of physical activity in good mental health.

The best studies randomly assign sedentary subjects to exercise and nonexercise groups and then measure psychological health before and

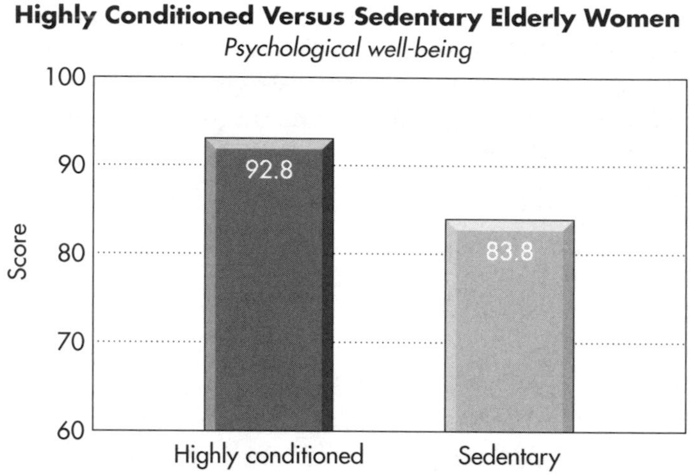

## Highly Conditioned Versus Sedentary Elderly Women
### Psychological well-being

FIGURE 18.2    When highly conditioned and sedentary elderly women (average age 73 years) were compared, general well-being scores were better in the fit women.

after in order to study the effects of adding regular exercise to the lifestyle. These studies are difficult and expensive to conduct, however, and few have followed large groups of people for long periods of time to allow drawing sound conclusions. Nonetheless, as will be emphasized in the rest of this chapter, growing evidence adds confirmation to the reports of superior mental health by physically active people, especially when the studies are long-term.

---

### Can physically fit and active people handle stress better than those who are inactive?

In general, physical fitness and activity are related to lower levels of cardiovascular arousal during and following mental stress. In some studies, physical fitness also helps buffer the body against the ill effects of mental stress.

---

When individuals are subjected to stressful situations, they experience an increase in heart rate, blood pressure, stress hormones, and nervous system activity. Researchers call this "cardiovascular reactivity" to mental stress. Researchers from Duke University have shown that in some susceptible individuals, cardiovascular reactivity can trigger heart attacks.

In the laboratory, scientists expose subjects to mentally challenging procedures such as matching geometric shapes and colors, playing color-word games, or solving arithmetic problems, attaching monetary rewards if a certain level of performance is reached. Studies have compared the cardiovascular reactivity to such laboratory tasks in highly fit versus unfit subjects or have followed people as they become fit to see if they improve their response.

Although not all researchers agree, exercise training is usually associated with a reduction in cardiovascular reactivity to mental stress. In one review of studies with some 1,500 subjects, aerobically fit individuals were found to have a significantly reduced reactivity response to a wide variety of stressful situations.

Reduction in reactivity to mental stress is felt to be important in day-to-day coping with work and life events. Exercise appears to be useful because as the individual adapts to the increase in heart rate, blood pressure, and stress hormones experienced during exercise, the body is strengthened and conditioned to react more calmly when the same responses are brought on during mental stress.

During the past 35 years, a large number of studies have shown that life events of all types (marriage, divorce, buying a house, losing one's job, moving to a new location, surgery for health problems, etc.) are significant stressors, leading to predictable physical and psychological health problems. Several studies have shown, however, that such life stress has less of a negative impact on the health of physically active individuals.

In a four-year study of 278 managers from 12 different corporations, for example, physical activity was found to have a buffering effect on the relationship between life events and illness. In other words, corporate managers who were active experienced fewer health problems from the stress they experienced than did inactive managers. Because it is not always practical or even possible to avoid many stressful life events, regular aerobic exercise may be one way to reduce the impact of stress on health.

In another study conducted by Dr. David Holmes, four groups of college students were identified: (1) high life stress, but highly physically fit; (2) high life stress, with low fitness levels; (3) low life stress, highly fit; and (4) low life stress, low levels of fitness. As shown in figure 18.3, psychological stress was related to high levels of physical illness, but only among individuals with low fitness levels. Students who had experienced high degrees of life stress but who were in good aerobic condition did not show higher levels of physical illness than did those who had not experienced high degrees of life stress.

**Physical Fitness Provides a Buffer Against Stress-Induced Health Problems**

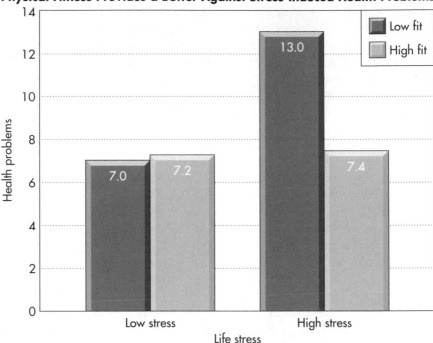

FIGURE 18.3   Students who experienced high stress but were also fit had low levels of sickness.

## Does regular exercise improve psychological well-being and mood?

Yes, this is a common and consistent finding, especially when the exercise is regular over the long term and the mood state is unfavorable to begin with.

Psychological mood state is often measured using validated questionnaires. In one questionnaire used by the U.S. Department of Health and Human Services, people are asked how they feel and how things have been going for them during the past month. Typical questions include "How have you been feeling in general?"; "Have you been bothered by nervousness or your 'nerves'?; "How happy, satisfied, or pleased have you been with your personal life?"; "Have you felt downhearted and blue?"; "Have you felt tired, worn out, used-up, or exhausted?" According to a point system, respondents are placed into classifications from "positive well-being" to "severely distressed."

Most studies have shown that psychological mood state is more favorable in active people and that it can be improved with regular exercise, especially when mood state is unfavorable to begin with. Figure 18.4 shows the results of one study of 36 physically inactive women who were randomly divided into walking and sedentary control groups. The walking group exercised at a brisk pace 45 minutes per day, five days per week, for 15 weeks, while the control group remained inactive.

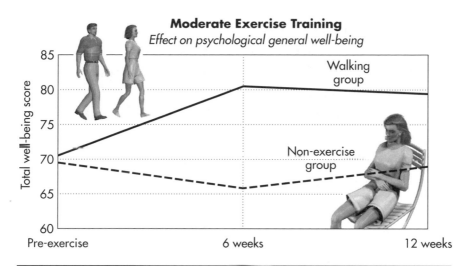

**FIGURE 18.4**  Regular brisk walking significantly improved psychological well-being.

Heart and lung fitness and psychological well-being were measured three times during the study to document how fast improvement took place. After just six weeks of exercise, the walkers improved their psychological well-being scores from an average of 70 (which indicates a stress problem) to 81 (indicating positive well-being), maintaining this throughout the 15-week study. The inactive control group did not show any significant change in their scores. Other psychological tests revealed that the walkers over time had higher energy levels, felt more relaxed and less tense or anxious, and sensed that life was more satisfying and interesting.

---

### Can regular exercise alleviate or prevent depression?

Most studies have shown that exercise is associated with reduced depression. The greatest improvements are seen in clinically depressed subjects who exercise frequently for several months.

---

A sizable proportion of Americans report feelings of depression, according to government researchers—about 7 percent of men and 11 percent of women during a given two-week period. Among elderly people, depression occurs in 15 percent of those living in the community, with higher rates found in nursing homes. The criteria for diagnosis of depression include

- changes in appetite and weight,
- disturbed sleep,
- fatigue and loss of energy,
- loss of interest or pleasure in usual activities,
- feelings of worthlessness, self-reproach, excessive guilt,
- suicidal thinking or attempts, and
- difficulty with thinking or concentration.

Depression may range in severity from mild symptoms to more severe forms. Recent studies have demonstrated that an overall increase in rates of major depression has occurred since World War II.

National surveys have suggested that sedentary adults are at much higher risk for feeling fatigue and depression than are those who are physically active. In one study of 1,536 Germans, the odds of being depressed were more than three times higher for sedentary versus physically active adults.

Many researchers have studied the link between exercise and depression. According to experts convened by the National Institute of Mental Health, most studies have shown that exercise is associated with reduced depression. Immediately following one bout of exercise, or in response to long-term regular exercise, a decrease in depression can be measured. The greatest improvements are seen in clinically depressed subjects who exercise frequently for several months.

In general, depressed patients when diagnosed are typically sedentary, and they then experience a sizable reduction in their depressive feelings when they initiate regular exercise. It has been proposed that exercise is as effective as group or individual psychotherapy or meditative relaxation in alleviating mild to moderate depression in patients. Dr. John Griest of the University of Wisconsin, for example, compared the effects of a running program against psychotherapy with depressed subjects. Running was found to be at least as effective as psychotherapy in alleviating moderate depression.

Anxiety, a condition characterized by apprehension, tension, or uneasiness, stems from the anticipation of real or imagined danger. This relatively normal feeling affects almost all people at some point in their lives. If the anxiety becomes excessive and unrealistic, however, it can interfere with normal functioning.

---

### Will I feel less tense if I exercise regularly?

Yes, both acute bouts of exercise (lasting at least 20 minutes) and chronic exercise training (for at least 10 months) have been related to reduced anxiety. The anxiety-reduction effect is seen with aerobic but not anaerobic (e.g., weight lifting) exercise.

---

Anxiety disorders, including various phobias, panic attacks, and obsessive-compulsive behavior, are the most prevalent of all mental health problems in the United States. Researchers measure anxiety by scoring responses to a variety of questions on tension, nervousness, self-confidence, indecisiveness, security, confusion, being worried, etc. Other measures of anxiety include blood pressure, heart rate, and skin responses or assessments of nervous system activity or muscular tension. Researchers have studied the effects of acute (before and after one bout) and chronic (before and after several weeks of training) exercise on anxiety.

One of the most frequently reported psychological benefits of exercise is a reduction in state anxiety (anxiety the subject feels "right now") following vigorous exercise, an effect that may last up to several hours.

One analysis of 104 studies of 3,048 subjects on the anxiety-reducing effects of exercise came to several conclusions, including these:

- Training programs usually need to exceed 10 weeks before significant changes in long-term anxiety occur.
- Exercise of at least 20 minutes' duration seems necessary to achieve reductions in both present and long-term anxiety.
- Reductions in both present and long-term anxiety occur after aerobic but not anaerobic (e.g., weight lifting) exercise training programs.

Figure 18.5 summarizes the results of one study involving 35 sedentary, mildly obese women (mean age 34 years) who were randomly assigned to exercise or nonexercise groups. Women in the exercise group walked briskly five times a week, 45 minutes per session, for 15 weeks, and experienced a significant reduction in anxiety relative to the nonexercise group. This study supports the idea that moderate

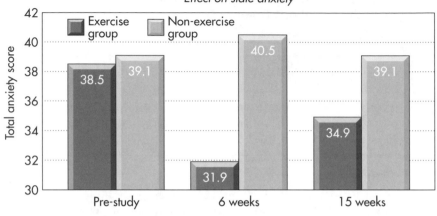

FIGURE 18.5    Regular brisk walking significantly lowered state anxiety in this randomized study.

aerobic exercise such as brisk walking is sufficient to reduce anxiety and tension.

---

### Can regular exercise improve self-esteem?

Yes, both aerobic and anaerobic exercise have been consistently related to improved self-esteem or self-concept.

---

Self-esteem or self-concept is defined as the degree to which individuals feel positive about themselves. Experts have identified self-esteem as the psychological variable with the greatest potential to be improved with exercise training, especially in those with initially low self-esteem. Even children and youth experience improved self-esteem with regular sport and physical activity.

In a study by Dr. James MacMahon of Stanford University, two hours per week of running and hard basketball led to significant improvements in psychological mood state and self-esteem in delinquent adolescent males incarcerated in juvenile detention facilities in Santa Clara County, California. The researchers concluded that vigorous aerobic exercise is of major psychological benefit to adolescents who exhibit aberrant behavior.

Weight training leads to measurable improvements in muscular strength and size, providing positive feedback that has been associated in many studies with an improvement in self-esteem. In one 12-week study of 60 women randomly assigned to weight training or brisk walking, body image improved in both groups, but more so in the weight lifters.

---

### Does regular exercise improve mental alertness and function?

For some aspects of mental function, exercise may be associated with small-to-moderate beneficial effects. More research is needed to sort out mixed results from current studies.

---

Many people report that they feel "mentally alert" shortly after a bout of exercise and that they can study with greater attentiveness. A large number of investigations have evaluated the effect of both acute and chronic exercise on cognition, using various tests involving word recall, memory searches, name retrieval, and the like.

Although much more research is needed, exercise does appear to have a small-to-moderate positive effect on mental function, especially when complex memory tasks are tested. Results indicate that memory and intellectual function may be improved during or shortly after an exercise session, as well as after long-term training. The mental function of elderly people, among all groups studied, appears to benefit the most from regular exercise. High versus low levels of physical fitness in old age have been related to improved cognition, especially for mental tasks that require rapid or effortful processing. Short-term training studies with elderly subjects have not shown an improvement in cognition, so regular exercise over the long term may be necessary before a positive effect is seen.

---

### How does physical activity improve psychological health?

There are at least six different theories that include an increased sense of mastery and self-confidence, social interaction, "time-out" from regular life stress, alterations in brain structure and chemicals, and elevation in body opiates that induce a good feeling. Depending on the individual, all of these factors together to one degree or another may contribute to the enhanced mental health of regular exercisers.

---

How and why exercise improves psychological health is a topic of active debate at present. Some of the more tenable theories can be grouped as follows:

• **Self-mastery:** As people start and then keep on with a regular exercise program (perceived by most as quite difficult), an increased sense of mastery and self-confidence can result. In other words, an "I can do it" attitude develops.

• **Social interaction:** Exercise is often done with others, leading to friendships, fun, and personal attention. Some researchers feel that this contributes to the mood elevation effects of exercise.

• **Time-out/distraction:** The contention here is that taking time out from the normal and stressful daily routine can result in mood elevation with some exercisers.

• **Improved brain fitness:** There is some thinking that aerobic exercise may increase blood flow and oxygen transport to the brain, inducing an elevation in mood state. Studies with animals suggest that permanent structural changes in the brain, including extra blood vessels and nerve endings, can result from regular exercise. Brain wave activity has also been found to be positively altered by exercise training or gains in physical fitness. Much more research is needed before the influence of exercise on the brain is fully understood.

• **Brain neurotransmitters:** Disturbances in the brain secretions of three brain chemicals or neurotransmitters—serotonin, dopamine, and norepinephrine—have been implicated in depression and other psychological disorders. Exercise may play a role in the treatment and prevention of depression by normalizing brain concentrations of these chemicals.

• **Body opioids:** Opiates have been used for centuries to relieve pain and induce euphoria. In 1975, researchers were successful in isolating chemicals from the body that were found to have "morphine-like" qualities. During vigorous exercise, the pituitary increases its production of one opiate called β-endorphin, leading to an increase in its concentration in the blood. Most researchers have found that β-endorphin does not increase unless the exercise is quite intense or the duration exceeds one hour. Although it is widely accepted by the exercising public that endorphins are responsible for exercise-induced euphoria, researchers disagree on whether or not exercise increases β-endorphin within the brain.

Depending on the individual, all of these factors together to one degree or another may contribute to the enhanced mental health of regular exercisers. Although there is some uncertainty about how exercise improves mental health, most experts agree that this is one of the strongest benefits of regular exercise.

Most mental health researchers have followed American College of Sports Medicine guidelines in their interventions, exercising their subjects for 30 to 60 minutes, three to five days a week, at a moderate to somewhat hard intensity. In other words, the same amount of exercise that is related to improved heart and lung fitness, and decreased risk of lifestyle diseases, also improves the mental fitness of the brain.

# REFERENCES

Barefoot, J.C., Larsen, S., von der Lieth, L., & Schroll, M. (1995). Hostility, incidence of acute myocardial infarction, and mortality in a sample of older Danish men and women. *American Journal of Epidemiology, 142,* 477-484.

Barefoot, J.C., & Schroll, M. (1996). Symptoms of depression, acute myocardial infarction, and total mortality in a community sample. *Circulation, 93,* 1976-1980.

Biddle, S. (1995). Exercise and psychosocial health. *Research Quarterly for Exercise and Sport, 66,* 292-297.

Chodzko-Zajko, W.J., & Moore, K.A. (1994). Physical fitness and cognitive functioning in aging. *Exercise and Sport Sciences Reviews, 22,* 195-220.

Cramer, S.R., Nieman, D.C., & Lee, J.W. (1991). The effects of moderate exercise training on psychological well-being and mood state in women. *Journal of Psychosomatic Research, 35,* 437-449.

Etnier, J.L., & Landers, D.M. (1995). Brain function and exercise: Current perspectives. *Sports Medicine, 19,* 81-85.

Hirschfeld, R.M.A., Keller, M.B., Panico, S., et al. (1997). The National Depressive and Manic-Depressive Association consensus statement on the undertreatment of depression. *Journal of the American Medical Association, 277,* 333-340.

Jiang, W., Babyak, M., Krantz, D.S., et al. (1996). Mental stress-induced myocardial ischemia and cardiac events. *Journal of the American Medical Association, 275,* 1651-1656.

Markovitz, J.H., Matthews, K.A., Kannel, W.B., Cobb, J.L., & D'Agostino, R.B. (1993). Psychological predictors of hypertension in the Framingham Study: Is there tension in hypertension? *Journal of the American Medical Association, 270,* 2439-2443.

McAuley, E., & Rudolph, D. (1995). Physical activity, aging, and psychological well-being. *Journal of Aging and Physical Activity, 3,* 67-96.

Nieman, D.C. (1995). *Fitness and sports medicine: A health-related approach.* Mountain View, CA: Mayfield.

Nieman, D.C., Warren, B.J., Dotson, R.G., Butterworth, D.E., & Henson, D.A. (1993). Physical activity, psychological well-being, and mood state in elderly women. *Journal of Aging and Physical Activity, 1*, 22-33.

North, T.C., McCullagh, P., & Tran, Z.V. (1990). Effect of exercise on depression. *Exercise and Sports Science Reviews, 18*, 379-415.

Petruzzello, S.J., Landers, D.M., Hatfield, B.D., Kubitz, K.A., & Salazar, W. (1991). A meta-analysis on the anxiety-reducing effects of acute and chronic exercise: Outcomes and recommendations. *Sports Medicine, 11*, 143-182.

Seward, B.L. (1994). *Managing stress: Principles and strategies for health and wellbeing.* Boston: Jones and Bartlett.

U.S. Department of Health and Human Services. (1996). *Physical activity and health: A report of the Surgeon General.* Atlanta: U.S. Department of Health and Human Services, Centers for Disease Control and Prevention, National Center for Chronic Disease Prevention and Health Promotion.

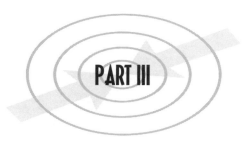

# PART III

# Physical Activity and the Life Cycle

This section of the book is devoted to physical fitness and activity issues related to children and youth, women, and those who are elderly. Concerns have been raised that our children and youth are not fit enough, are overweight, and are being passed by as their parents participate in the current adult fitness movement. In chapter 19, these concerns will be addressed. During the last three decades, there has been a dramatic increase in the number of women participating in both recreational and competitive sports. With this increase has come a much better understanding of how men and women differ and how they compare in their ability to exercise and compete, as will be reviewed in chapter 20. A key ingredient to healthy aging, according to many experts who study elderly people, is regular physical activity. Of all age groups, those who are elderly have the most to gain by being active, as will be highlighted in chapter 21.

# Chapter 19

# CHILDREN AND YOUTH

U.S. youth do not engage in physical activity, within or outside physical education, sufficient to develop cardiovascular endurance. Our youth are, therefore, at risk of developing a myriad of diseases associated with sedentary lifestyles.

### Dr. Charles T. Kuntzleman

There is a perceived "fitness crisis" among American children and youth. This has been a cause for grave concern among politicians and parents alike, prompting countless workshops, conventions, editorials, and government expert panels.

The general viewpoint is that American children and youth are less healthy, active, and physically fit than is recommended. The recent concern over youth fitness started in the mid-1950s when Dr. Hans Kraus, a noted orthopedic physician, reported data showing that the fitness scores of U.S. youth were not as good as the scores of European youth.

When President Eisenhower became aware of the report after widespread public outcry, he called for a special White House Conference on the topic. As a result, the President's Council on Physical Fitness and Sports was formed.

Several national surveys during the 1980s and 1990s have provided more data showing that there is reason to be worried about youth fitness:

• **Young people are increasingly overweight.** Among those 6 to 17 years of age, 22 percent (about 10 million) are overweight, an increase of six percentage points from the late 1970s. A high proportion of overweight youth end up obese as adults. About half of obese school-age children become obese adults, and more than 80 percent of obese adolescents remain obese into adulthood.

- **Only half exercise vigorously.** Only about one-half of U.S. young people (ages 12 to 21 years) regularly participate in vigorous physical activity, while one-fourth get none at all. Only one in three students in grades 5 through 12 takes physical education daily, with this proportion falling to one in five among high school students. Even for students taking physical education, observers have noted that less than 10 percent of class time is spent in moderate-to-vigorous physical activity.

- **Girls exercise less than boys.** Activity levels of girls are below those of boys and tend to drop sharply as age or grade in school increases.

- **Upper-body strength is poor.** The upper-body strength is poor for many children and youth. For example, for girls ages 9 to 17, about half cannot perform more than one pull-up. Among boys ages 6 to 12, 40 percent cannot do more than one pull-up, while 25 percent cannot do any.

- **Aerobic fitness is poor.** Heart and lung fitness is lower than recommended for many young people. About half of girls 6 to 17 years of age, and 60 percent of boys ages 6 to 12, cannot run a mile in less than 10 minutes.

- **Many have disease risk factors.** About 12 percent of children and youth ages 12 to 17 smoke, with the proportion rising to 25 percent among high school seniors. Close to one in three children and adolescents has serum cholesterol levels that exceed 170 mg/dl, the level deemed "acceptable" by the National Cholesterol Education Program. A national survey by the Centers for Disease Control revealed that 63 percent of adolescents have two or more of five major risk factors for chronic disease. Risk factors tend to cluster and show tracking from childhood and adolescence to adulthood, meaning that every attempt should be made while a person is young to bring risk factors under control.

For physically active adults, there are numerous health benefits, as described in this book. Does physical activity improve the health of children and youth and carry over into adulthood? Do young people respond differently to exercise than adults, and should their activity programs be adapted as a result? Information to answer these questions will be reviewed in this chapter, but the reader should understand that less evidence exists for the young in comparison to what is currently available for adults.

Most experts feel that children and youth need daily physical activity to keep fit and healthy. Researchers have noted, however, that when children engage in physical activity, they mix very short bursts of intense activity with easy-to-moderate activity. Children often find it difficult to exercise at a constant pace for 20 or more minutes, and would rather engage in play and sporting activities of a more stop-and-go nature.

For children, parents and teachers are urged to provide many opportunities for play and simple sports. Enjoyment has been identified as the major reason why children engage in physical activity. Physically active parents and role models provide support for children to be active. The American Academy of Pediatrics has emphasized that children need active play, good physical education programs, parental involvement, and generally active lifestyles rather than specific vigorous exercise training.

The Centers for Disease Control and Prevention (CDC) in 1997 released guidelines urging schools to help young people get active and stay active. Various CDC recommendations encouraged school officials to

- provide recess activities such as jumping rope,
- not withhold activity as punishment,
- emphasize areas such as dancing and walking to encourage life-long habits, and
- tell parents to be physically active with their kids.

The CDC guidelines state that physical activity programs for young people are most likely to be effective when they:

- Emphasize enjoyable participation in physical activities that are easily done throughout life.
- Offer a variety of noncompetitive and competitive activities suitable for different ages and abilities.
- Give young people the skills and confidence they need to be physically active.
- Promote physical activity through a comprehensive school health program with links to the community.

Judy Young, executive director of the National Association for Sports and Physical Education, says that children probably need more activity than adults. Overall, there is so little research on children and exercise training that few other guidelines can be stated with certainty.

---

## Should teenagers follow the same activity guidelines recommended for adults?

Most experts recommend that teenagers follow adult physical activity guidelines.

---

In 1993, an international group of experts sponsored by 13 scientific, medical, and governmental organizations submitted guidelines on physical activity for teenagers. Two guidelines were recommended:

• All adolescents should be physically active nearly every day. The activity can be a part of play, games, sport, work, transportation, recreation, physical education classes, or planned exercise with the family or community. Adolescents should engage in a variety of physical activities, and these should be enjoyable and should involve most of the major muscle groups. The experts agreed that this would help reduce the risk of obesity and promote healthy bones. According to Dr. James Sallis, who chaired the consensus conference, "This is consistent with adult recommendations to engage in 30 minutes of daily activities of moderate intensity." Studies show that most adolescents meet this guideline, getting about 60 minutes per day of some type of physical activity, most of it outside of school. Unfortunately, during adolescence, time spent by both girls and boys in physical activity declines, and the decline continues into adulthood.

• Teenagers should pursue vigorous exercise for 20 minutes or more each session at least three times a week. Only about two-thirds of adolescent males and one-half of females meet this guideline. Examples of recommended activities include brisk walking, jogging, stair climbing, basketball, racquet sports, soccer, dance, lap swimming, skating, weight training, lawn mowing, cross-country skiing, and cycling. The consensus was that the more vigorous exercise should enhance psychological health, increase high-density lipoprotein cholesterol, and increase cardiorespiratory fitness.

---

## Do children and youths respond to aerobic exercise programs similarly to adults?

Before they reach physical maturity, children and youth can improve aerobic fitness in response to training, but to a smaller degree than in adults.

---

Most researchers have reported that the cardiorespiratory systems of children and youth respond to regular aerobic exercise in a fashion somewhat similar to that seen in adults. There are a few differences, however.

Dr. Thomas Rowland of the Baystate Medical Center in Springfield, Massachusetts, has shown that children can improve aerobic fitness after training but that the increase is less than for adults. In one study of 37 boys and girls, ages 11 to 13 years, 12 weeks of regular aerobic training improved $\dot{V}O_2$max by 6.5 percent, about half what adults typically experience. Dr. Rowland concluded that several factors may be responsible for this: (1) children often have high aerobic fitness levels to begin with; (2) adults may train more effectively than children; and (3) the bodies of children may lack the ability to adapt and respond fully to regular exercise.

There are some other important differences between children and adults. Children have smaller hearts, lungs, and blood volumes. The heart of a child cannot pump out as much blood per minute of exercise, so there is a lower oxygen delivery to the working muscles. $\dot{V}O_2$max does not fully develop until late adolescence.

Children have a larger body surface area than adults when calculated per unit of body mass. As a result, the smaller the child, the greater is the risk of excessive heat loss. This is particularly important when the child exercises in water, which can draw the body heat from the child very quickly, leading to hypothermia (i.e., low body temperature). To prevent hypothermia, children who swim or play in the water should be encouraged to leave the water periodically and to avoid cold lakes and streams.

Children as compared to adults have a less well-developed sweating capacity. They also produce more heat during activities such as running or vigorous sports play and can experience a faster increase in body temperature when dehydrated. These differences put children at risk for heat-related illness during long-term exercise in the heat. Researchers urge that children drink fluids frequently and avoid excessive exercise in the heat.

---

### Is it safe for children and youths to lift weights?

Yes, but before physical maturity is reached, weight training should be moderate and supervised.

---

For many years, weight training was not recommended for children and adolescents for two reasons. First, heavy weight lifting was thought to interfere with bone growth and to promote bone and joint injury. Secondly, it was claimed that weight training was not effective in children before the time of puberty.

Most studies now support weight training as both safe and effective for children and youths. Still, the American Academy of Pediatrics has cautioned that children and adolescents should avoid intensive weight lifting, power lifting, and bodybuilding until they are about 15 years of age. Moderate weight lifting by children should be under adult supervision to decrease the risk of injury. Weight training is recommended two or three times a week for 20 to 30 minutes a session, and should be part of an overall comprehensive program designed to increase total fitness.

According to most experts, children can improve strength with appropriate weight training by about 15 to 30 percent. The rise in strength is not usually related to any measurable increase in muscle size, however. Instead, improvements in nerve and muscle cell interactions occur, augmenting strength.

---

### Should teenagers have a medical exam before participating in competitive sports?

There is growing support for the idea that adolescent athletes should have a thorough medical exam that checks for heart defects before playing competitive sports.

---

There have been a disturbing number of sudden deaths in young competitive athletes in recent years. Fatal heart problems strike about 12 young athletes yearly, most of them of high school age. Dr. Barry Maron of the Minneapolis Heart Institute Foundation, a leading expert in this area, has found that most of these deaths are precipitated by vigorous exercise and are due to a wide variety of heart defects, most commonly hypertrophic cardiomyopathy (an abnormal thickening of the heart muscle of the left ventricle).

The question has been whether thorough physical exams could help identify those at risk of sudden death. In most cases of sudden death, athletes had been given physicals and were cleared to compete. The cost for more sensitive tests that would detect heart defects is up to $2,000 a screening. That's not cost effective given the nearly six million scholastic athletes in the United States and the fact that the tests are not usually covered by health insurance.

Nonetheless, heart disease experts are calling for standardized nationwide exams for young athletes to prevent sudden deaths on the playing field. New guidelines, recommending the use of relatively inexpensive procedures that can pick up many of the heart defects, have been issued by the American Heart Association. Experts urge that parents and teachers look for these signs and symptoms in susceptible young athletes:

- Fainting episodes
- Sudden chest pain
- High blood pressure
- High or uneven heart rate
- Family history of heart disease
- Family history of sudden, unexplained death

---

## Does regular physical activity help children and youths avoid obesity?

Obesity in children and youths has been linked to physical inactivity.

---

Most studies suggest that obese children and youth are less physically active than their leaner peers. However, whether the obesity causes the inactivity or vice versa is still a matter of debate.

For example, in one study of 77 preschool children in the southeast of England, low levels of physical activity were linked to high levels of body fat. However, the researchers led by Dr. Peter Davies of Cambridge stressed that "it is impossible to determine absolutely whether reduced activity causes an increase in body fat or that a higher level of body fatness restricts, and therefore reduces activity."

It does make sense, however, that long-term inactivity on the part of children would increase the risk of gaining extra body fat. Indeed, this was the finding of a group of researchers from Boston University who followed about 100 children for several years. In this study, children with low levels of physical activity gained more body fat over the years than did more active children.

Dr. Oded Bar-Or from Canada feels that "programs longer than one year are more efficacious than shorter programs. Lifestyle activities (e.g., walking to and from school) appear to have a more lasting effect than regimented activities (e.g., calisthenics or jogging)."

As noted earlier in this chapter, adults can often trace their problems with obesity to their childhood and adolescence. Obviously, if children and youth are helped to keep active and lean, the risk of obesity later on in life can be reduced. Also, obesity during childhood has been linked to other disease risk factors such as high blood pressure and cholesterol. If children avoid obesity, other risk factors can more easily be brought under good control.

Children and youth spend an inordinate amount of time when not in school watching television, viewing videos, or playing computerized games. There has been an ongoing debate as to whether or not these sedentary habits are linked to obesity and whether they prevent children and youth from getting recommended amounts of physical activity. Although not all researchers agree, most have shown that the link is real and that such sedentary pursuits should be limited to less than one or two hours a day in order to allow sufficient time for more strenuous activities.

---

*Are children who exercise at less risk of developing disease?*
Although many other lifestyle factors are involved, regular physical activity does appear to help keep some risk factors under control, especially in children and youth who are in greatest need of improvement.

---

Many studies have shown that heart disease, cancer, and other chronic diseases are linked to the lifestyles of people, and that these behaviors are learned in childhood and adolescence and become established by young adulthood. Experts also agree that the health habits that teenagers tend to adopt are related to how acceptable the behavior is believed to be among their peers (i.e., peer pressure).

In that health habits are embedded within the very fabric of American life, most experts recommend that prevention should be aimed at young people, especially through school programs. Large-scale studies have shown that it is possible to work through the school systems to increase the amount of physical activity children get throughout the day. For example, in the Child and Adolescent Trial for Cardiovascular Health (CATCH), over 5,000 children were followed for three years, with efforts directed toward enhancing school physical and health education, as well as school lunch programs.

Results showed that students improved both the amount and intensity of their physical activity in response to the CATCH program and also reduced their intake of dietary fat. Blood pressure and cholesterol, however, did not change as a result of the lifestyle improvements. The researchers urged that "it may be more important for this age group to demonstrate the ability to modify nutrition and physical activity behaviors in ways leading to lifetime health habits rather than to reduce immediate risk levels." In other words, "success" should be defined more by the positive change in health habits than by risk factors.

Most studies show that compared to physically inactive children and youth, those who exercise regularly have lower resting blood pressures and more favorable blood lipid profiles. However, it is difficult to know whether this is due to the exercise or to other lifestyle habits. When sedentary children and youth initiate exercise programs, there may be some improvement in blood pressure and lipids, but usually only among those with initially high levels. Often other positive changes contribute to this effect, including decreases in body and dietary fat.

As reviewed in the chapter on osteoporosis, peak bone mineral density is reached by young adulthood. The great majority of bone buildup occurs during adolescence. One of the most valuable health benefits of regular and vigorous exercise early in life is that a higher peak bone mineral density is achieved, reducing the risk for early osteoporosis later on in life.

Experts recommend that weight-bearing activities (e.g., most team and dual sports, running) are better than weight-supported activities such as swimming and cycling in building strong bones among the youth. Short, intense daily activity is better than prolonged activity done infrequently, and activities that increase muscle strength, like weight lifting, should be promoted. All of the body's muscle should be exercised in order to provide benefit to all of the bones.

---

### Are active youth less likely to smoke and drink alcohol than inactive youth?

There is some support for the viewpoint that physically active young people tend to smoke less than inactive youth. However, other health habits have not been consistently tied to exercise.

---

This has been a difficult question to answer. Many people believe that sport and exercise keep children and youth out of mischief and away from smoking and using alcohol and drugs. There is some support from the Centers for Disease Control and Prevention for the idea that adolescents involved in interscholastic sports and vigorous exercise smoke less than those exercising little. The link of exercise to other positive health habits among children and youth has not been consistently established.

A team of researchers from the University of Pittsburgh followed 1,245 adolescents for three years, studying the link between physical activity and the onset of such unhealthy behaviors as cigarette smoking, alcohol consumption, and the carrying of weapons. Highly active teenage girls were half as likely to start smoking during the study than were those who had low levels of physical activity. Highly active teenage boys, in contrast, tended to start smoking at the same rate as their less active peers, and were twice as likely to start drinking alcohol. No connection between physical activity and weapon carrying was found.

Dr. Deborah Aaron, who headed up the study, cautions that while it "would be appealing to assume, and in fact is a well-accepted notion, that adolescents who are physically active are less likely to engage in poor health behaviors," little support for this notion actually exists. Nonetheless, Dr. Aaron does find encouragement in the connection between physical activity and fewer new smokers among the teenage girls, and urges that "participation in women's high school athletic programs may reduce the growing problem of the initiation of female smoking."

Data from the 1990 Youth Risk Behavior Survey on 11,631 high school students suggest that low physical activity is tied to several other negative health behaviors including cigarette smoking, marijuana use, lower fruit and vegetable intake, greater television viewing, and failure to wear a seat belt. However, physical activity was not linked to other behaviors such as cocaine use, sexual activity, physical fighting, self-perception of weight, and alcohol consumption among the males. The researchers urged that future studies examine whether programs aimed at increasing physical activity in youth can improve overall health behavior.

---

### Will an active child be an active adult?

Although there is some tracking of exercise habits into adulthood, many people become inactive when making the transition from student to young adult.

---

This has been an attractive hypothesis: Help children and youth adopt regular exercise habits when young, and they should keep exercising throughout their lifetime. Unfortunately, this theory has not held up too well.

Most studies have shown that physical activity drops sharply during late adolescence and early adulthood. In one long-term study of some 5,000 men and women, a 50 percent decline in the amount of physical activity was measured between the ages of 18 and 37 years. In other words, there appears to be little carryover of exercise habits from youth to adulthood. Experts state that these findings point strongly to a need for physical activity promotion programs aimed toward young adults as they make the transition from student to employee.

# REFERENCES

Aaron, D.J., Dearwater, S.R., Anderson, R., Olsen, T., Kriska, A.M., & LaPorte, R.E. (1995). Physical activity and the initiation of high-risk health behaviors in adolescents. *Medicine and Science in Sports and Exercise, 27,* 1639-1645.

Anderssen, N., Jacobs, D.R., Sidney, S., et al. (1996). Change and secular trends in physical activity patterns in young adults: A seven-year longitudinal follow-up in the Coronary Artery Risk Development in Young Adults Study (CARDIA). *American Journal of Epidemiology, 143,* 351-362.

Centers for Disease Control and Prevention. (1997). Guidelines for school and community programs to promote lifelong physical activity among young people. MMWR 46, No. RR-6.

Davies, P.S.W., Gregory, J., & White, A. (1995). Physical activity and body fatness in pre-school children. *International Journal of Obesity, 19,* 6-10.

Falk, B., & Tenenbaum, G. (1996). The effectiveness of resistance training in children. A meta-analysis. *Sports Medicine, 22,* 176-186.

Kuntzleman, C.T. (1993). Childhood fitness: What is happening? What needs to be done? *Preventive Medicine, 22,* 520-532.

Lowry, R., Kann, L., Collins, J.L., & Kolbe, L.J. (1996). The effect of socioeconomic status on chronic disease risk behaviors among US adolescents. *Journal of the American Medical Association, 276,* 792-797.

Luepker, R.V., Perry, C.L., McKinlay, S.M., et al. (1996). Outcomes of a field trial to improve children's dietary patterns and physical activity. The Child and Adolescent Trial for Cardiovascular Health (CATCH). *Journal of the American Medical Association, 275,* 768-776.

Maron, B.J., Shirani, J., Poliac, L.C., Mathenge, R., Roberts, W.C., & Mueller, F.O. (1996). Sudden death in young competitive athletes: Clinical, demographic, and pathological profiles. *Journal of the American Medical Association, 276,* 199-204.

Myers, L., Coughlin, S.S., Webber, L.S., Srinivasan, S.R., & Berenson, G.S. (1995). Prediction of adult cardiovascular multifactorial risk status from childhood risk factor levels: The Bogalusa Heart Study. *American Journal of Epidemiology, 142,* 918-924.

Pate, R.R., Heath, G.W., Dowda, M., & Trost, S.G. (1996). Associations between physical activity and other health behaviors in a representative sample of US adolescents. *American Journal of Public Health, 86*, 1577-1581.

Riddoch, C.J., & Boreham, C.A.G. (1995). The health-related physical activity of children. *Sports Medicine, 19*, 86-102.

Rowland, T.W., & Boyajian, A. (1995). Aerobic response to endurance exercise training in children. *Pediatrics, 96*, 654-658.

Sallis, J.F., & Patrick, K. (1994). Physical activity guidelines for adolescents: Consensus statement. *Pediatric Exercise Science, 6*, 302-314.

Simons-Morton, B.G., KcKenzie, T.J., Stone, E., Mitchell, P., Osganian, V., Strikmiller, P.K., Ehlinger, S., Cribb, P., & Nader, P.R. (1997). Physical activity in a multiethnic population of third graders in four states. *American Journal of Public Health, 87*, 45-50.

Simons-Morton, B.G., Taylor, W.C., Snider, S.A., Huang, I.W., & Fulton, J.E. (1994). Observed levels of elementary and middle school children's physical activity during physical education classes. *Preventive Medicine, 23*, 437-441.

Troiano, R.P., Flegal, K.M., Kuczmarski, R.J., Campbell, S.M., & Johnson, C.L. (1995). Overweight prevalence and trends for children and adolescents. The National Health and Nutrition Examination Surveys, 1963 to 1991. *Archives of Pediatric and Adolescent Medicine, 149*, 1085-1091.

U.S. Department of Health and Human Services. (1996). *Physical activity and health: A report of the Surgeon General.* Atlanta: U.S. Department of Health and Human Services, Centers for Disease Control and Prevention, National Center for Chronic Disease Prevention and Health Promotion.

# Chapter 20

# SPECIAL ISSUES FOR WOMEN

As every runner knows, running is about more than just
putting one foot in front of the other; it is about our
lifestyle and who we are.

**Joan Benoit Samuelson**

Since the time of the ancient Greeks and Romans, women have been
viewed more for their beauty than their athletic ability. The athletic
arena has traditionally been a male domain. When it came to vigorous
physical labor, however, women were expected to join right in—a role
they continue to perform in Third World countries.

It wasn't long ago that women were thought to be too fragile to
compete. Women were first allowed to participate in the 1912 Olympics,
and some events such as the women's marathon were added only in
1984. At the end of the 800-meter race in the 1928 Olympics, the *New York
Times* reported, "The cinder track was strewn with wretched damsels in
agonized distress." No women's race longer than 200 meters would be
run until 32 years later.

Today, more and more sports are available to women, and there is a
push worldwide to ensure equity for women in sport. The Atlanta
Olympic Games, for example, involved a record number of women
(3,779, including 280 on the U.S. team) and sports for women (21).

And women are proving that they are capable of feats once thought
impossible for the "weaker sex." At the 1984 Olympic Games in Los
Angeles, Joan Benoit won the gold medal in the first-ever Olympic
marathon race event for women. Her time was 2 hours and 24 minutes,
a standard that would have won 11 of the previous 20 men's Olympic
marathons. In 1988, Paula Newby-Fraser completed the Hawaiian
Ironman Triathlon, comprising a 2.4-mile sea swim, a 111-mile cycle
ride, and a 26-mile run, in 9 hours and 1 minute, just 30 minutes or 6
percent slower than the time of the male winner. Only 10 men were

ahead of her that year. During the 1990s, women runners and swimmers from China have stunned the world with their commanding performances. For example, Wang Junxia set a world record for the 10,000-meter race in September of 1993 by running a time of 29 minutes and 31 seconds, shattering the old record by 42 seconds. Wang's time would have bettered that of all male runners prior to 1949.

The gap between the best men and women athletes has shrunk sharply during the past quarter century. In the Boston Marathon, for example, the difference in winning times for men and women diminished from 54 minutes in 1972 to about 16 minutes in 1995. However, the gender performance gap in many endurance events has now stabilized, largely because the quick gains following the loosening of social restraints have run their course. Figure 20.1 summarizes world record times in the 5,000-meter run for men and women. Notice that women started late in racing 5,000 meters and quickly began to narrow the gender gap, but then stalled during the mid-1980s.

More women are exercising today than ever before. Women now engage in strenuous recreational and competitive physical activities

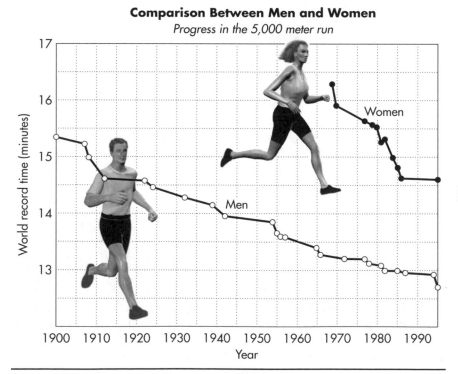

**Comparison Between Men and Women**
*Progress in the 5,000 meter run*

FIGURE 20.1    Women started late in racing 5,000m; the gender gap narrowed quickly but has now stabilized.

once deemed socially unacceptable for them. Women of the 1960s were concerned about the stigma of getting big muscles from exercise and about whether their femininity would be marred. Today interests center on the same fitness and performance issues that concern men.

Despite these trends, the best national surveys still show that more women than men are physically sedentary. And men are more likely than women to engage in vigorous physical activity and muscle-strengthening activities like weight training. There still is much more room for progress, and research is needed to more clearly define how the genders differ in their responses to exercise training.

---

## Can women get as fit as men?

Although there are some important differences between the sexes in size, strength, and other aspects of physiology, both men and women show expected improvements in physical fitness through regular training.

---

At puberty, testosterone secretion in males increases, leading to larger bones and increased muscle mass. In females, estrogen secretion increases, broadening the pelvis, stimulating breast development, and increasing the amount of fat in the thigh and hip areas. These unique sex differences continue into adulthood, and largely explain why men and women differ in size, strength, and athletic performance.

When the top female runners in the world are compared with their male counterparts, race times are 9 to 15 percent slower over all distances. This gap is not expected to decrease, largely because males and females differ in several important areas related to physical fitness.

• **Heart and lung fitness:** Women have less hemoglobin in their blood than men do, reducing the amount of oxygen that can be delivered to working muscles. Women also tend to have more body fat, less skeletal muscle, and smaller lungs and hearts. Together, these factors mean that women have a lower $\dot{V}O_2$max than men (25 percent lower on average when nonathletes are compared) and tend to perform at a lower level in aerobic sports such as running, cycling, swimming, and rowing. When women and men train at the same intensity, duration, and frequency, both show expected improvements in $\dot{V}O_2$max. Men, however, usually start and end at higher levels. Elite female athletes have $\dot{V}O_2$max values that exceed those of most men, but these values still fall 8 to 12 percent below those of elite male athletes.

• **Muscle strength and size:** The average woman has about half the upper-body strength of men and one-fourth the lower-body strength. In the weight room, women can experience strength gains with regular training, but increase in muscle size is less than what is seen in most men. Of course there are some female bodybuilders who have more muscle size and definition than most untrained men. There are few such women, however, and the best female bodybuilders cannot compare in muscle mass to the best male bodybuilders. In general, women have less muscle and more fat than men, and this is an important reason for the gap in performance times between the genders.

---

### Do women and men get the same health benefits from exercise?

Although fewer studies have been conducted on women than on men, in general the two sexes appear to obtain similar health benefits from regular physical activity.

---

The leading causes of death among women are quite similar to those for men:

| Women (% of all deaths) | Men (% of all deaths) |
|---|---|
| 1. Heart disease (34.0%) | 1. Heart disease (31.6%) |
| 2. Cancer (22.6%) | 2. Cancer (24.1%) |
| 3. Stroke (8.2%) | 3. Stroke (5.1%) |
| 4. COPD* (4.2%) | 4. COPD (4.7%) |
| 5. Pneumonia/influenza (4.1%) | 5. Accidents (5.2%) |
| 6. Accidents (2.8%) | 6. Pneumonia/influenza (3.3%) |
| 7. Diabetes (2.8%) | 7. Diabetes (2.0%) |

*COPD = chronic obstructive pulmonary disease (e.g., emphysema).

There are a few differences, however. Before menopause, women have very low rates of heart disease. After menopause, the rates increase steeply, and by the eighth decade, there is no difference in this regard between men and women. For cancer, women most commonly get breast cancer, while men contend with prostate cancer. However, for both sexes, lung cancer is the most common cancer killer, followed by breast cancer for women, prostate cancer for men, and then colorectal cancer for both.

Most of the early studies showing that regular physical activity provided protection from heart disease, cancer, stroke, diabetes, and other chronic diseases were conducted with men. Only recently have women been studied, and more research is needed to provide a clear answer to the question whether or not women realize the same health benefits as men do from exercise.

In previous chapters of this book, many available studies on women have been highlighted. For example, a study of some 1,200 women in Seattle showed that regular moderate exercise decreased the risk of heart attacks by 50 percent. In Rhode Island, sedentary women were found to have double the risk for coronary heart disease as compared to physically active women. In Copenhagen, risk for stroke was 1.5 times greater for physically inactive versus active women.

A large study of over 40,000 women in Iowa showed that regular phyisical activity reduced risk of death from all causes by 30 percent. Women who participated in vigorous exercise experienced a 40 percent reduction in risk of death.

In general, these and other studies indicate that women gain the following health benefits from regular physical activity:

- Lower risk of coronary heart disease and stroke
- Lower risk of breast and colon cancer, and possibly various reproductive cancers
- Decreased risk of diabetes
- Improved bone density and a decreased risk for osteoporosis
- Improved long-term weight control
- Improved psychological well-being
- Enhanced body function in old age
- Decreased risk of high blood pressure
- Improved blood lipid profile

---

### Can too much exercise be harmful to women?

For some female athletes, the pressure to keep body weight low and be successful can lead to heavy training and disordered eating, loss of the menstrual period, and thinning of the bones, a syndrome called the "female athlete triad."

---

It was in 1972 that President Richard Nixon signed into law Title IX, the federal legislation mandating equal opportunities for collegiate female athletes. Funding has also increased to support girls playing high school sports. By 1995-1996, high school girls' sport participation rose to 2.4 million, compared with 3.6 million for boys. Basketball, outdoor track, volleyball, softball, and soccer are the sports with the most young female participants.

The pressure to succeed in competitive sports has led some women to train heavily while eating less than recommended in order to achieve low body weights and high performance levels. Under these stresses, some women may lose their menstrual periods, a condition termed amenorrhea. If the amenorrhea is experienced long enough, the estrogen levels in the woman's body drop, causing the bones to lose mineral mass, leading to early osteoporosis. This syndrome of heavy exercise and undereating, amenorrhea, and osteoporosis is called the female athlete triad (see figure 20.2).

Typically, only about 2 to 5 percent of the female population have amenorrhea. This proportion, however, can climb to 50-65 percent in some athletic groups, especially female runners and ballet dancers.

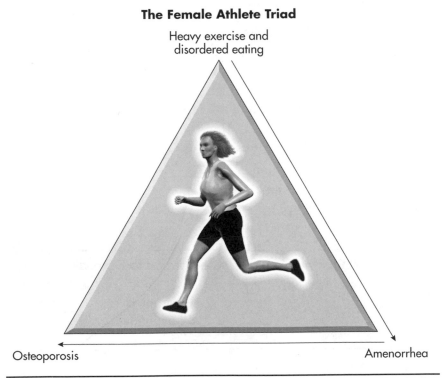

**The Female Athlete Triad**

Heavy exercise and
disordered eating

Osteoporosis                                    Amenorrhea

FIGURE 20.2    Some female athletes train too hard and eat too little. This can lead to loss of the menstrual period and bone mineral density.

Women who participate in sports that emphasize low body weight are at special risk (e.g., gymnasts, divers, cheerleaders, figure skaters, and aerobic dancers). Close to half of female runners who train 80 or more miles a week are amenorrheic, compared to only 5 to 10 percent of runners who are moderate in their training. In female athletes with amenorrhea, the density of bones is 10 to 30 percent lower than normal, and risk of stress fractures in the bones of the legs and feet is high.

It appears that heavy amounts of exercise can actually disrupt the release of certain hormones from the brain that are needed by the ovaries to go through a normal and full cycle. Also, when the female athlete does not eat enough, the body goes into a semistarvation mode, interrupting the normal release of hormones that drive the menstrual cycle.

Although the percentage of athletic women who eat poorly is not known for certain, estimates from experts range from 30 to 65 percent. With the disruption in menstrual periods, estrogen levels drop to levels experienced by women after menopause, leading to a rapid loss of bone mass.

All women who stop menstruating or who menstruate irregularly because of their exercise program are urged to see a physician, start eating more while exercising less, increase calcium intake to 1,500 milligrams a day, and in some cases receive estrogen/progesterone replacement therapy. With these changes, the menstrual period often returns, and bone mass is built back up to near normal levels for many but not all female athletes.

---

### Is exercise safe for a pregnant woman and her baby?

In general, maintenance of regular physical activity during pregnancy helps keep the mother fit and healthy, causes no harm to the growing fetus, and may improve the birthing experience.

---

Earlier in this century, pregnant women were urged to reduce physical activity and stop working, especially during the later stages of pregnancy. Exercise was thought to increase the risk of early labor by stimulating uterine activity.

At the other end of the continuum are some female athletes who continue training throughout their pregnancy. Ingride Kristiansen, the famous runner from Norway, for example, ran to the day of labor and delivered a healthy baby boy. Five months later, she ran a 2:27 marathon, and then a few months later, a 2:24, and within two years she held the world records for the 5K, 10K, and marathon.

*Runner's World* reported the story of a woman who ran up to 40 miles a week throughout her pregnancy. Nine days before giving birth, she completed a marathon race. The day before giving birth to a healthy baby boy, she competed in a 24-hour race, running 62.5 miles.

Many athletes have the attitude expressed by Dr. Joan Ullyot, a physician and marathon runner who has observed, "Gazelles run when they're pregnant. Why should it be any different for women?" These types of stories have concerned many experts and physicians who provide health care for women.

Moderate amounts of exercise during pregnancy are recommended for the health and fitness of the mother and baby. One large-scale study of some 2,000 women in Missouri showed that those who largely avoided exercise during pregnancy were more likely to give birth to very low birth weight infants (who are more prone to sickness and death).

In another study of some 400 pregnant women, aerobic exercise throughout pregnancy led to fewer discomforts later on. A few studies even suggest that fit mothers gain less unnecessary body fat during pregnancy, experience shorter labor, and have fewer cesarean-section births.

Debate still centers on whether or not intense and prolonged exercise by the pregnant mother can cause harm to the growing fetus. Concern has been expressed that during heavy exertion, body temperature may rise to high levels while blood flow, glucose supply, and oxygen delivery to the fetus may be decreased, affecting normal development.

In 1985, the American College of Obstetricians and Gynecologists (ACOG) released guidelines for exercise during pregnancy. They took a cautious approach, urging that pregnant women exercise moderately for only 15 minutes at a time, keeping the heart rate below 140 beats per minute. These guidelines caused an outcry among some experts who claimed they were too conservative. In one review of the medical literature, researchers concluded that exercise performed for up to 40 to 45 minutes, three times a week at a heart rate of up to 140 to 145 beats per minute, did not appear to adversely affect the mother or fetus.

In 1994, ACOG released their new guidelines, removing the heart rate recommendation. According to ACOG, "There are no data in humans to indicate that pregnant women should limit exercise intensity and lower target heart rates because of potential adverse effects." However, ACOG did urge that regular, moderate exercise is sufficient to derive health benefits and that pregnant women should listen to their bodies, stop exercising when fatigued, and not exercise to exhaustion.

Does strenuous exercise reduce the ability of the mother to provide breast milk for her baby? Little research has been conducted in this area, but in one study conducted at the University of California in Davis, vigorous exercise for up to 1.5 hours a day had no negative effect on ability to lactate. Exercise during lactation is recommended to help the mother build up fitness and muscle tone.

---

### Do different phases of the menstrual cycle affect a woman's ability to exercise?

Although some women report that premenstrual symptoms interfere with ability to exercise, researchers have been unable to link this with actual changes in the body. Female athletes report that they can rise above their feelings when necessary to compete, and have set world records during all phases of the cycle.

---

In surveys, one-third and up to two-thirds of female athletes report that their ability to exercise is not negatively affected during any phase of the menstrual cycle. Up to one-fourth report that performance is hindered during the premenstrual phase and the first few days of menstrual flow, with an improvement during the immediate postmenstrual days. Many women link premenstrual symptoms (PMS) such as fluid retention, weight gain, and mood changes with decreases in ability to exercise.

Scientists have studied whether there are actual physiological explanations for these reports by women athletes. Changes in many body functions do occur throughout the normal menstrual cycle, but researchers have been unable to associate menstrual cycle phase with problems in athletic performance.

Experts point out that world records have been set during all phases of the menstrual cycle. Joan Benoit Samuelson's period was due the day of the 1984 Olympic Marathon, and she won. "If I'm focused on a big race and expecting PMS or my period, the adrenaline from my excitement takes over and wipes out any negative feelings. My period becomes inconsequential—a peripheral event."

Can regular exercise reduce PMS symptoms? Very few studies exist in this area. Researchers at Duke University exercised women for three months and reported that aerobic exercise decreased PMS symptoms, especially depression. Women who become serious runners report milder PMS and better moods than women who remain physically inactive. Most current studies have serious design flaws, and better research is needed to determine whether decreases in PMS symptoms are due to exercise or other factors such as weight loss, dietary changes, expectations, or improved self-esteem.

---

### Can exercise help relieve the symptoms of menopause?

Most experts view exercise as a valuable adjunct to hormone replacement therapy in controlling symptoms and problems experienced during menopause.

---

Menopause, defined as the woman's final menstrual period, occurs at an average age of 52 years. Several symptoms and problems are common among women during the time of menopause, due in part to hormonal changes, the aging process, and poor lifestyle habits. Hormone replacement therapy (both estrogen and progestogen) relieves the hot flushes, helps prevent bone loss, reduces cardiovascular risk, and improves mood and sleep quality.

Exercise is a valuable adjunct to hormone replacement therapy for a woman around the time of menopause. Exercise can help prevent bone loss, counter loss of muscle strength, reduce cardiovascular risk, improve mood and sleep quality, and help prevent weight gain.

Exercise, however, has not been shown to relieve hot flushes or other menopause symptoms. In one large study of 2,000 Australian-born women, no link between physical activity and menopausal symptoms was seen.

## REFERENCES

American College of Sports Medicine. (1997). The female athlete triad. *Medicine and Science in Sports and Exercise, 29,* i-ix.

Bam, J., Noakes, T.D., Juritz, J., & Dennis, S.C. (1997). Could women outrun men in ultramarathon races? *Medicine and Science in Sports and Exercise, 29,* 244-247.

Barrett-Connor, E. (1997). Sex differences in coronary heart disease. Why are women so superior? *Circulation, 95,* 252-264.

Clapp, J.F., & Little, K.D. (1995). Effect of recreational exercise on pregnancy weight gain and subcutaneous fat deposition. *Medicine and Science in Sports and Exercise, 27,* 170-177.

Dueck, C.A., Matt, K.S., Manore, M.M., & Skinner, J.S. (1996). Treatment of athletic amenorrhea with a diet and training intervention program. *International Journal of Sport Nutrition, 6,* 24-40.

Guthrie, J.R., Smith, A.M., Dennerstein, L., & Morse, C. (1994). Physical activity and the menopause experience: A cross-sectional study. *Maturitas (MWN)*, *20*, 71-80.

Kushi, L.H., Fee, R.M., Folsom, A.R., Mink, P.J., Anderson, K.E., and Sellers, T.A. (1997). Physical activity and mortality in postmenopausal women. *Journal of the American Medical Association, 277*, 1287-1292.

Lebrun, C.M. (1993). Effect of the different phases of the menstrual cycle and oral contraceptives on athletic performance. *Sports Medicine, 16*, 400-430.

Lovelady, C.A., Nommsen-Rivers, L.A., McCrory, M.A., & Dewey, K.G. (1995). Effects of exercise on plasma lipids and metabolism of lactating women. *Medicine and Science in Sports and Exercise, 27*, 22-28.

Rencken, M.L., Chesnut, C.H., & Drinkwater, B.L. (1996). Bone density at multiple skeletal sites in amenorrheic athletes. *Journal of the American Medical Association, 276*, 238-240.

Samuelson, J.B., & Averbuch, G. (1995). *Running for women*. Emmaus, PA: Rodale Press.

Schramm, W.F., Stockbauer, J.W., & Hoffman, H.J. (1996). Exercise, employment, other daily activities, and adverse pregnancy outcomes. *American Journal of Epidemiology, 143*, 211-218.

Shangold, M.M. (1996). An active menopause: Using exercise to combat symptoms. *The Physician and Sportsmedicine, 24* (7), 30-36.

Sternfeld, B. (1997). Physical activity and pregnancy outcome: Review and recommendations. *Sports Medicine, 23*, 33-47.

Sternfeld, B., Quesenberry, C.P., Eskenazi, B., & Newman, L.A. (1995). Exercise during pregnancy and pregnancy outcome. *Medicine and Science in Sports and Exercise, 27*, 634-640.

Wells, C.L. (1996). Physical activity and women's health. *Physical Activity and Fitness Research Digest*, Series 2 (5), 1-8.

Wilmore, J.H., & Costill, D.L. (1994). *Physiology of sport and exercise*. Champaign, IL: Human Kinetics.

# Chapter 21

# THE ELDERLY

You only have one body. There are no retreads.

Hulda Crooks, centenarian and mountain climber

Although Americans idolize youth and spare no expense to regain it, the United States is now regarded by experts as an "aging society." In colonial times, for instance, the average age of the population was 16 years. Today it is 33 years, and by 2030 it will grow to 42 years.

During the last century, dramatic improvements in life expectancy (i.e., the expected number of years of life at a given age) have been realized in many countries worldwide. In the United States, for example, life expectancy has increased from 47 to nearly 76 years during the past nine decades and is expected to exceed 82 years by the year 2050. In 1900, only 40 percent of Americans lived beyond age 65, a proportion that has now doubled to 80 percent. The fastest-growing minority in the United States is the "very old" (85-and-older population), a group that is projected to expand from 3.1 million in 1990 to approximately 17.7 million by the year 2050.

The key issue, caution scientists who study aging, is that of quality of life. The National Center for Health Statistics has estimated that 15 percent of the average American's life, or about 12 years, is spent in an "unhealthy" state (i.e., impaired by disabilities, injuries, and/or disease). Among those reaching age 65, it is predicted that 5 of their remaining 17 to 18 years, on average, will be unhealthy ones.

Nearly 85 percent of elderly people have one or more diseases or health problems. Between 4 and 11 percent of people over the age of 65 years have some form of senile dementia, especially Alzheimer's disease. The most frequently occurring health problems among elderly people are these:

- Arthritis (48 percent of elderly persons)

- High blood pressure (36 percent)
- Heart disease (32 percent)
- Hearing impairments (32 percent)
- Orthopedic impairments (19 percent)
- Cataracts (17 percent)
- Diabetes (11 percent)
- Visual impairments (9 percent)

The aging process varies widely between people and is influenced by both lifestyle and genetic factors. Experts on aging feel that humans could live to age 115 to 120 years on a regular basis if both the lifestyle and genetic backgrounds were optimal. Several people have lived to 120 years of age or more. Arthur Reed of Oakland, California, lived to be 124 years of age. Shigechigo Isumi of Japan died in 1986 at the age of 121 years. Mary Thompson of Orlando, Florida, died in 1996 at the age of 120 years.

About 6 in 10 Americans want to live to be 100 years old, according to a survey by the Alliance for Aging Research. And two-thirds believe that they have some control over how long they will live, with 9 out of 10 willing to adopt a more positive outlook, eat more nutritious food, or exercise regularly to achieve that goal. The greatest fears about growing old involve living in a nursing home (64 percent of people surveyed) and getting Alzheimer's disease (56 percent).

Exercise, diet, smoking, and other health habits have a strong effect in improving both the length and quality of life. Dr. Lester Breslow of UCLA, for example, in his famous study of over 6,000 people in the San Francisco Bay Area, showed a dramatic difference in death rates between those who followed seven simple health habits (never smoked, moderate alcohol intake, daily breakfast, no snacking, seven to eight hours of sleep per night, regular exercise, ideal weight) and those who did not. Those who followed all seven health habits had much lower death rates, and it was estimated that they would live nine years longer than those who did not practice any of the health habits. In addition, those adhering to the healthy lifestyle habits were only half as likely to have had disabilities that kept them from work or that limited day-to-day activities.

A key ingredient to healthy aging, according to many gerontologists (i.e., those who study aging), is regular physical activity. Of all age groups, people who are elderly have the most to gain by being active. The risk for many diseases and health problems common in old age (e.g., cardiovascular disease, cancer, high blood pressure, depression, osteoporosis, bone fractures, and diabetes) is decreased with regular physical activity.

Regular exercise can also decrease body fat and increase muscle strength, as well as improve aerobic fitness. Fit elderly people can better take care of themselves and engage in the common activities of life. Elderly people who exercise regularly report that they sleep better, are less vulnerable to viral illnesses, and have a better quality of life than their sedentary friends.

Yet national surveys indicate that only about 37 percent of older men and 24 percent of older women participate in physical activities three or more times a week for 30 minutes or more. This is less than for any other age group.

Interestingly, many of the changes that come with aging are similar to those that occur during long-term bed rest and weightlessness. These include a decrease in heart and lung function, an increase in body fat, a decrease in muscle size and strength, and loss of bone mineral density. As will be emphasized in the paragraphs to follow, much of the deterioration that was once attributed to aging is instead now linked to physical inactivity. Nonetheless, the aging process is real, and although remarkable amounts of body function and fitness can be attained in old age, inevitably aging always wins. The goal is to push back frailty to a very small part of the life experience, or as Ashley Montagne has urged, "to die young as late in life as possible."

---

### Is exercise as effective in helping older people stay lean as it is for younger people?

Yes, but unusual attention to diet and exercise habits is necessary.

---

Studies show that body fat approximately doubles between the ages of 20 and 65 years. During middle age, extra fat often is gained around the stomach and trunk areas, which is especially harmful to long-term health. The increase in body fat usually occurs at the same time that muscle and bone mass is decreasing. This ends up being a vicious cycle in that the resting metabolic rate drops as a result, making further gains in body fat more likely.

The energy metabolism research team at the Jean Mayer U.S. Department of Agriculture Human Nutrition Research Center on Aging at Tufts University, Boston, has determined that older people lose some of their ability to "waste" the excess calories taken in after overeating. Older people need to be aware that they may not burn off surplus energy as easily as they did when they were younger.

To compensate, those who are elderly should avoid overeating and should exercise daily. Studies of athletic elderly people have shown that low body fat is possible in old age but comes only in those who are unusually vigilant in their exercise and diet habits (i.e., combining daily activity with moderate eating).

---

## Will a weight-training program help older people gain strength?

Yes, studies show that it is never too late to improve muscle strength and size through weight training, and that elderly people who do so can greatly improve function and life quality. However, to keep muscle strength and size near the levels of young adulthood requires a lifetime of whole-body resistance exercise.

---

Muscular strength in most people is maintained to about 45 years of age, but falls by about 5 to 10 percent per decade thereafter. The average person will lose about 30 percent of his or her muscle strength and 40 percent of muscle size between the ages of 20 and 70 years. This loss in muscle mass appears to be the major reason that strength is decreased in those who are elderly. In older people, muscle weakness may decrease the ability to accomplish the common activities of daily living, leading to dependency on others. Also, reduced leg strength may increase the risk of injury through falling.

A growing number of studies have now clearly shown that elderly persons, even into their 90s, are capable of increasing muscle size and strength in response to weight training. Overall, studies suggest that the decline in strength and muscle mass with increase in age can be lessened by appropriate resistance training. Many experts feel that strength training by people who are elderly can greatly improve the quality of their lives and that increased muscle size and strength are among the chief benefits of exercise in old age.

The problem is that many middle-aged and elderly people are not motivated to train with weights. Calisthenics in the home as well as work activities around the home can be used, but these must be demanding in order to maintain muscular size and strength. A lifetime of vigorous exercise is necessary to keep all of the body's muscles in good shape.

Many researchers who have evaluated the effects of aging on the cardiorespiratory system have focused on maximal aerobic fitness, or $VO_2$max. The ability of the body to take in oxygen, transport it, and use it to burn fuel is seen by many as the single best measure to represent the changes that occur in the body with aging.

---

## Can aerobic training improve heart and lung fitness even in old age?

Aerobic fitness declines by about 8 to 10 percent per decade during adulthood. Regular aerobic training can help people of all ages attain aerobic fitness levels equal to those of untrained people much younger than themselves.

---

$\dot{V}O_2$max normally declines 8 to 10 percent per decade for both males and females after 25 years of age. About half of this decrease has been related to people's exercising less and getting fatter as they age.

Despite this, at any given age, people can have a much higher $\dot{V}O_2$max if they exercise vigorously and keep lean. Master athletes who are 65 to 75 years of age can have the $\dot{V}O_2$max of young sedentary adults and are capable of performing at levels once thought unattainable.

Warren Utes of Illinois, for example, in 1991 at the age of 70 set an age-group world record of 38:24 for the 10K race. Sixty-year-old Luciano Acquarone of Italy ran a 2:38 marathon, a pace of 6 minutes a mile, while Derek Turnbull of New Zealand ran 5 kilometers in 16:39 at the age of 65. Evy Palm at the age of 49 ran a half-marathon in 1:12:36 in Holland—a time regarded as one of the top-rated age-graded performances of all time. In 1996, 71-year-old John Keston of England ran a world best marathon time of 3:01 for those over the age of 70. His goal is to break 3 hours for the marathon, a threshold once thought impossible for septuagenarians. Tiny Riley ran 5 kilometers in 48:35, a U.S. age-group mark for women. At age 91, she's the oldest woman in the U.S. record books.

However, even among athletes who exercise vigorously throughout their lifetimes, $\dot{V}O_2$max still declines at a rate similar to that of sedentary individuals (albeit at a much higher absolute level). Some studies have demonstrated that the rate of decline may be lessened for up to 20 years because of regular, vigorous endurance exercise, but if subjects are followed long enough, $\dot{V}O_2$max will start falling at normal or accelerated rates.

Researchers from Ball State University studied former elite distance runners over a 22-year period and found that regardless of how much they trained, all lost aerobic fitness. Those who trained the hardest were able to push back the rate of decline a bit, but this worked best for middle-aged, not elderly runners.

In other words, there are no convincing data at this time to show that the age-related decrease in aerobic fitness can be prevented through regular endurance exercise training. The aging process is real, and several changes in the body, including a decrease in the ability of the heart to pump blood at a high rate and the capacity of the muscles to use oxygen, are linked to the age-related decline in $VO_2$max.

The bottom line is that at any given age, athletes who exercise vigorously can be fitter than their sedentary counterparts, but because of the aging process, will be less fit than younger athletes. Studies have confirmed that peak performance for men is achieved in their 20s for all running and swim events (e.g., 23 years for sprinting and 28 for marathon running). It should be emphasized, however, that most studies support the fact that untrained people even in their eighth decade of life have not lost the ability to adapt to aerobic exercise training. In other words, it is never too late to improve from an untrained to a trained state.

Figure 21.1 shows the results of a study in which untrained elderly women (average age of 73 years) were analyzed for aerobic fitness, compared to athletic peers who were active in senior games competitions, and then randomized to walking and control groups. Notice that the elderly athletic women had aerobic fitness levels two-thirds higher than those of the sedentary women. The elderly women who began walking for 37 minutes a day, five days a week, improved their fitness 13 percent in just 12 weeks, an increase similar to that seen for young adults. However, they still fell far below the levels of their athletic peers who had been trained intensely for 11 years and were competing in race

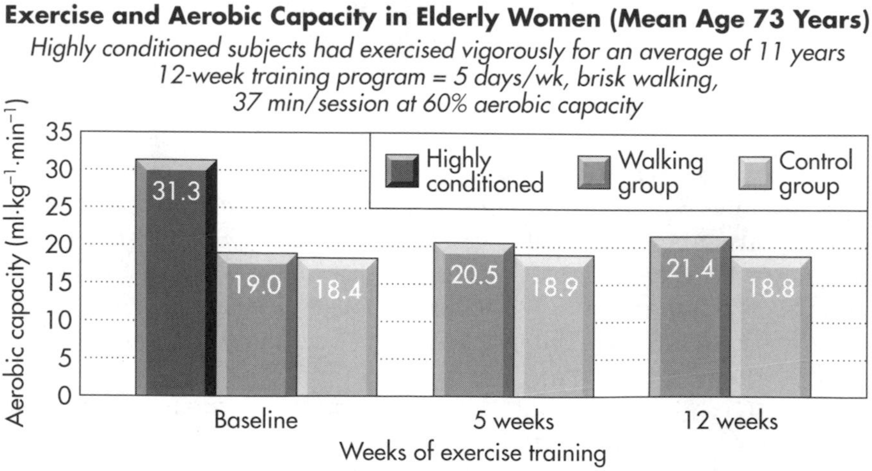

**Exercise and Aerobic Capacity in Elderly Women (Mean Age 73 Years)**

*Highly conditioned subjects had exercised vigorously for an average of 11 years*
*12-week training program = 5 days/wk, brisk walking,*
*37 min/session at 60% aerobic capacity*

FIGURE 21.1    Brisk walking improved fitness 13%, but fell far below that of athletic peers.

events. The main points here are that women even in their 70s can be trained and that they can be unusually fit if highly dedicated to their exercise programs.

---

### Are there any special guidelines for aerobic exercise programs for elderly people?

The same basic aerobic exercise programs used for young adults can be applied to persons who are elderly. However, to avoid injuries, elderly people starting an exercise program are urged to progress more slowly and cautiously.

---

Although earlier studies suggested that older individuals were not as responsive to aerobic training as their younger counterparts, there is now a growing consensus that gains in aerobic fitness are similar for elderly people, albeit at a lower level. In general, the same basic exercise programs used for young adults can be applied to elderly individuals, but with an emphasis on greater caution and slower progression.

There is some concern about exercise-induced injury rates among elderly people. While walking appears safe and effective for this group, jogging may lead to unusually high injury rates. Elderly persons appear to be more fragile and more prone to joint injury during such aerobic activities as jogging or aerobic dance. Activities such as walking, swimming, or stationary cycling may be preferable.

A thorough medical exam with a treadmill-electrocardiographic (EKG) test is recommended for elderly individuals prior to starting an exercise program. People who are elderly often have special medical considerations that should be cleared first with a doctor.

---

### Do active people live longer?

Yes, nearly all studies have shown that death rates for all causes combined are lower in physically active and fit people when compared to those who largely avoid exercise. In practical terms, middle-aged adults who are physically active gain on average about two years of life.

---

As described earlier in this chapter, life expectancy is defined as the average number of years of life expected for people of a certain age. For example, babies born today are expected to live 76 years on average, while 65-year-olds are expected to live an average of another 18 years. Life span, on the other hand, refers to the maximum age thought to be obtainable by a given animal species. For humans, the life span is thought to be about 115 to 120 years; for Indian elephants, about 70 years; for domestic cats, 28 years; and for house mice, 3 years.

Most experts feel that exercise has little effect on the life span but has a powerful impact on life expectancy. The majority of studies have shown that physically active people have less heart disease and cancer, and lower death rates overall, than those who are physically sedentary. According to Dr. I-Min Lee of Harvard University, "The most active or fit individuals experience mortality rates that are, perhaps, one-quarter to one-half lower than the rates among those least active or fit."

Although some confusion exists, there is a growing sentiment among researchers that most of the benefits come from accumulating 30 minutes or more of moderate-intensity physical activity on most days of the week. However, additional health and longevity benefits come when people put in a greater amount of more intensive exercise.

Findings from the Harvard Alumni Health Study, for example, suggest that increasing amounts of physical activity are associated with decreased mortality, especially when the activity is conducted vigorously (e.g., uphill brisk walking). In general, life expectancy was found to be about two years greater in those exercising 2,000 calories per week. In practical terms, this improvement in life expectancy can be attained by brisk walking a minimum of 8 to 10 miles a week. Although the extra time linked to physical activity may not seem to be much, researchers remind us that if cancer were completely removed from the United States, the average person would live about two years longer. In other words, regular physical activity has the same effect on life expectancy for the average person that elimination of cancer would have.

Data from the Cooper Institute for Aerobics Research have shown that the least fit of men and women are about twice as likely to die as their fit counterparts. In fact, as shown in figure 21.2, low fitness turned out to be one of the strongest risk factors for death rates from all causes. As emphasized by Dr. Steven Blair, who headed up the study, "Becoming fit has a similar effect on reduction in mortality to stopping smoking."

Dr. Lauren Lissner of Göteborg University in Sweden followed a group of some 1,400 women for 20 years, and found that death rates from all causes were cut by more than half among those who were regularly physically active. According to Dr. Lissner, "This study confirms that physical inactivity is one of the strongest predictors of mortality and suggests that maintenance of leisure-time activity levels is an important health promoter in aging populations."

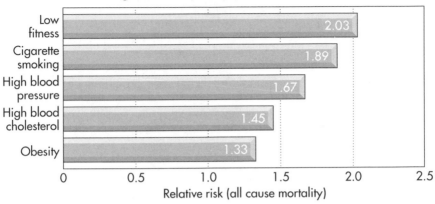

**Relative Risk of Death From All Causes**
Among 25,341 men, Cooper Institute for Aerobics Research

FIGURE 21.2   Low fitness is a leading risk factor for early death.

## A CASE STUDY

The data that I have been gathering for over 12 years on Mavis Lindgren illustrate nicely the key issues in this chapter. Mavis was sedentary most of her life until age 63, when she began walking for her health. After a few months of slow progression, she built up to walking and then jogging 25 to 30 miles a week, a routine she faithfully kept for seven years.

At the age of 70, in response to a challenge laid down by her physician son, she increased her training to 40 to 50 miles per week and ran her first marathon. Mavis found that she enjoyed the challenge of marathon running and the attention it brought her. Nineteen years later, at the age of 89, Mavis had completed 73 marathons and was still running 40 to 50 miles a week. During this time she became the oldest woman ever to race to the top of Pike's Peak in Colorado and to finish the New York City Marathon.

Figure 21.3 plots the race times for these marathons, as well as the results of 10 treadmill $\dot{V}O_2$max tests that were conducted on Mavis between the ages of 77 and 89. There are several interesting points to be made, especially considering the information this chapter has presented.

• Between the ages of 80 and 83, Mavis' $\dot{V}O_2$max fell rapidly, and then plateaued despite maintenance of a training schedule of 40 to 50 miles a week. $\dot{V}O_2$max decreased 34 percent between the ages of 77 and

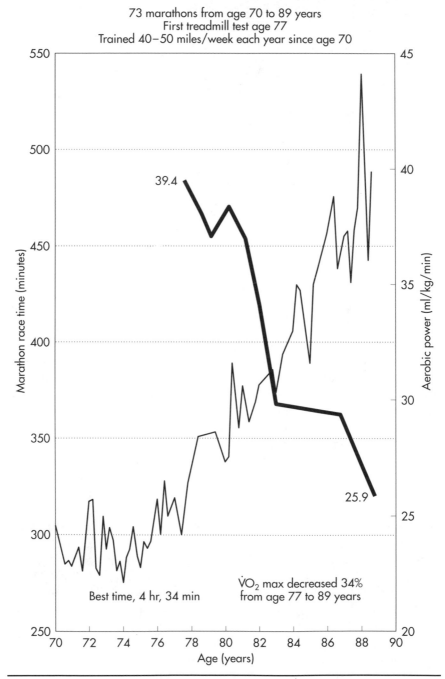

**FIGURE 21.3**   Though much fitter than her peers, Mavis' V̇O₂max and performance still fell in her 80s.

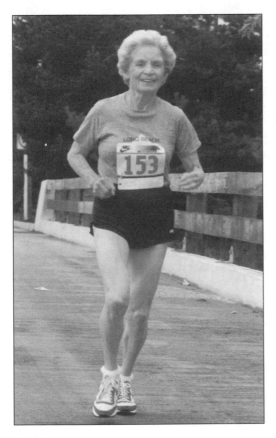

89; this was during a period when Mavis' marathon race times increased by about two-thirds. There are probably several reasons for this loss of aerobic fitness and racing ability, including effects due to the aging process itself and a decline in ability to sustain a high training intensity despite unusually high motivation.

- Between the ages of 77 and 80, Mavis' $\dot{V}O_2$max averaged about 38 ml $\cdot$ kg$^{-1}$ $\cdot$ min$^{-1}$, an aerobic fitness level equal to that of untrained women in their 20s. Despite significant decreases in her aerobic power since age 77, Mavis still enjoys the $\dot{V}O_2$max of a woman about 25 years younger than herself.

Mavis has demonstrated that it is never too late to start exercising and that an unusually high $\dot{V}O_2$max is possible even in old age when there is a motivation to engage in large amounts of exercise.

# REFERENCES

Blair, S.N., Kampert, J.B., Kohl, H.W., et al. (1996). Influences of cardiorespiratory fitness and other precursors on cardiovascular disease and all-cause mortality in men and women. *Journal of the American Medical Association, 276,* 205-210.

Blair, S.N., Kohl, H.W., Barlow, C.E., et al. (1995). Changes in physical fitness and all-cause mortality: A prospective study of healthy and unhealthy men. *Journal of the American Medical Association, 273,* 1093-1098.

Green, J.S., & Crouse, S.F. (1995). The effects of endurance training on functional capacity in the elderly: A meta-analysis. *Medicine and Science in Sports and Exercise, 27,* 920-926.

Jackson, A.S., Beard, E.F., Wier, L.T., et al. (1995). Changes in aerobic power in men, ages 25-70 yr. *Medicine and Science in Sports and Exercise, 27,* 113-120.

Jackson, A.S., Wier, L.T., Ayers, G.W., Beard, E.F., Stuteville, J.E., & Blair, S.N. (1996). Changes in aerobic power of women, ages 20-64 yr. *Medicine and Science in Sports and Exercise, 28,* 884-891.

Lee, I-M., Hsieh, C-C., & Paffenbarger, R.S. (1995). Exercise intensity and longevity in men: The Harvard Alumni Healthy Study. *Journal of the American Medical Association, 273,* 1179-1184.

Lee, I-M., & Paffenbarger, R.S. (1996). Do physical activity and physical fitness avert premature mortality? *Exercise and Sports Science Reviews, 24,* 135-169.

Lissner, L., Bengtsson, C., Björkelung, C., & Wedel, H. (1996). Physical activity levels and changes in relation to longevity: A prospective study of Swedish women. *American Journal of Epidemiology, 143,* 54-62.

Nelson, M.E., Fitarone, M.A., Morganti, C.M., et al. (1994). Effects of high-intensity strength training on multiple risk factors for osteoporotic fractures: A randomized controlled trial. *Journal of the American Medical Association, 272,* 1909-1914.

Nieman, D.C. (1995). *Fitness and sports medicine: A health-related approach.* Mountain View, CA: Mayfield.

Paffenbarger, R.S., Hyde, R.T., Wing, A.L., et al. (1993). The association of changes in physical activity level and other lifestyle characteristics with mortality among men. *New England Journal of Medicine, 328,* 538-545.

Pollock, M.L., Carroll, J.F., Graves, J.E., et al. (1991). Injuries and adherence to walk/jog and resistance training programs in the elderly. *Medicine and Science in Sports and Exercise, 23,* 1194-1200.

Pollock, M.L., Mengelkoch, L.J., Graves, J.E., Lowenthal, D.T., Limacher, M.C., Foster, C., and Wilmore, J.H. (1997). Twenty-year follow-up of aerobic power and body composition of older track athletes. *Journal of Applied Physiology, 82,* 1508-1516.

Province, M.A., Hadley, E.C., Hornbrook, M.C., et al. (1995). The effects of exercise on falls in elderly patients: A preplanned meta-analysis of the FICSIT trials. *Journal of the American Medical Association, 273,* 1341-1347.

Rogers, M.A., & Evans, W.J. (1993). Changes in skeletal muscle with aging: Effects of exercise training. *Exercise and Sports Science Review, 21,* 65-102.

Trappe, S.W., Costill, D.L., Vukovich, M.D., Jones, J., & Melham, T. (1996). Aging among elite distance runners: A 22-yr longitudinal study. *Journal of Applied Physiology, 80,* 285-290.

Warren, B.J., Nieman, D.C., Dotson, R.G., et al. (1993). Cardiorespiratory responses to exercise training in septuagenarian women. *International Journal of Sports Medicine, 14,* 60-65.

Yusuf, H.R., Croft, J.B., Giles, W.H., et al. (1996). Leisure-time physical activity among older adults: United States, 1990. *Archives of Internal Medicine, 156,* 1321-1326.

# Chapter 22

# THE BENEFITS OF REGULAR EXERCISE

*The greatest health benefits from an increase in activity appear to occur when very sedentary persons begin a regular program of moderate intensity, endurance-type activity.*

**Dr. William L. Haskell, Stanford University School of Medicine**

Exercise is a powerful medicine quite unlike any pill available. At the beginning of the book, I described a "magical elixir" that lengthened the span and quality of life, decreased risk of heart disease, diabetes, and colon cancer by nearly half, alleviated mental anxiety and depression, improved muscle tone and heart function, and lowered blood pressure.

Well, such a potion does exist, but time and effort are involved—two barriers that can make regular physical activity a bitter pill to swallow for some. Nonetheless, for those willing to make the sacrifice, this health-saving nostrum brings intoxicating benefits with few side effects.

This book has chronicled just how effective physical activity can be in both preventing and treating the wide variety of ailments that plague modern men and women. Throughout recorded history, philosophers, world leaders, and physicians have extolled the virtues of regular exercise. Despite this pervasive belief in the goodness of exercise, only within the last few decades have scientific data emerged to warm the hearts of fitness enthusiasts and persuade even the strongest critics.

As emphasized by Dr. William Haskell of the Stanford University School of Medicine, the greatest health benefits come when very sedentary people begin and maintain a regular program of moderate physical activity. In other words, from a public health viewpoint, getting the most physically inactive portion of Americans to become moderately active will lead to the strongest health gains.

Perhaps one of the strongest points to take away from this book is that the sedentary life followed by one in four Americans is extremely risky and is to be avoided at all costs. The Centers for Disease Control and Prevention has estimated, for example, that sedentary living causes about one-third of deaths due to coronary heart disease, colon cancer, and diabetes and that about 250,000 deaths a year in the United States are related to physical inactivity.

To avoid the health pitfalls of the sedentary life, the Centers for Disease Control and Prevention and the American College of Sports Medicine urge that every adult accumulate 30 minutes or more of moderate-intensity physical activity (not necessarily all at one time) on most, preferably all, days of the week. While aerobic exercise is most important for health benefits, keeping the muscles toned and strong improves life quality and the ability to accomplish the common tasks of everyday life, especially in old age.

This amount of physical activity, 30 minutes or more nearly every day, appears to be a basic level that can lead to improvements in health and prevention of disease. However, as illustrated in figure 22.1, additional health and fitness benefits can be experienced as the amount and intensity of exercise increase, a point that was highlighted in the 1996 Surgeon General's report on physical activity and health.

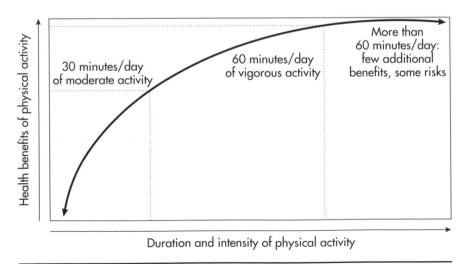

FIGURE 22.1    Most health benefits come from moderate amounts of activity.

Debate still centers around the optimal amount of physical activity needed for health. Dr. Per Olaf Åstrand, a leading European pioneer in exercise physiology, feels that at least 60 minutes a day of physical activity, not necessarily vigorous or all at the same time, combined with at least two or three 30-minute vigorous exercise sessions each week, is required. Other experts agree that the human body needs more than an hour a day of physical activity to stay in good health. They reason that our ancestors did much more, and we should not be surprised that we need at least an hour a day of moderate-to-vigorous physical activity to stave off disease.

In this book, the evidence for and against potential benefits of physical activity was reviewed. For some areas of health and disease, a large amount of data from studies was available to enable one to state with surety that regular exercise is beneficial or protective. In other areas, much more research is needed before firm conclusions can be reached. Table 22.1 summarizes the various health benefits discussed in this book, with a rating given for each one to indicate just how sure scientists are that exercise is related.

TABLE 22.1

## The Health Benefits of Regular Physical Activity[1]

| Physical activity benefit | Surety rating |
|---|---|
| **Fitness of body** | |
| Improved heart and lung fitness | ★ ★ ★ ★ |
| Improved muscular strength/size | ★ ★ ★ ★ |
| **Cardiovascular disease** | |
| Coronary heart disease prevention | ★ ★ ★ ★ |
| Regression of atherosclerosis | ★ ★ |
| Treatment of heart disease | ★ ★ ★ |
| Prevention of stroke | ★ ★ |
| **Cancer** | |
| Prevention of colon cancer | ★ ★ ★ ★ |
| Prevention of breast cancer | ★ ★ |
| Prevention of uterine cancer | ★ ★ |
| Prevention of prostate cancer | ★ ★ |
| Prevention of other cancers | ★ |
| Treatment of cancer | ★ |

*(continued)*

TABLE 22.1 *(continued)*
# The Health Benefits of Regular Physical Activity[1]

| Physical activity benefit | Surety rating |
|---|---|
| **Diabetes** | |
| Prevention of NIDDM | ★ ★ ★ ★ |
| Treatment of NIDDM | ★ ★ ★ |
| Treatment of IDDM | ★ |
| Improvement in diabetic life quality | ★ ★ ★ |
| **Osteoporosis** | |
| Helps build up bone density | ★ ★ ★ ★ |
| Prevention of osteoporosis | ★ ★ ★ |
| Treatment of osteoporosis | ★ ★ |
| **Arthritis** | |
| Prevention of arthritis | ★ |
| Treatment/cure of arthritis | ★ |
| Improvement in life quality/fitness | ★ ★ ★ ★ |
| **Low back pain** | |
| Prevention of low back pain | ★ ★ |
| Treatment of low back pain | ★ ★ |
| **Asthma** | |
| Prevention/treatment of asthma | ★ |
| Improvement in life quality | ★ ★ ★ |
| **Infection and immunity** | |
| Prevention of the common cold | ★ ★ |
| Improvement in overall immunity | ★ ★ |
| Slower progression of HIV to AIDS | ★ |
| Improvement in life quality of HIV-infected | ★ ★ ★ |
| **Cigarette smoking** | |
| Improvement in success in quitting | ★ ★ |
| **Blood cholesterol/lipoproteins** | |
| Lower blood total cholesterol | ★ |
| Lower LDL-cholesterol | ★ |
| Lower triglycerides | ★ ★ ★ |
| Raised HDL-cholesterol | ★ ★ ★ |
| **High blood pressure** | |
| Prevention of high blood pressure | ★ ★ ★ ★ |
| Treatment of high blood pressure | ★ ★ ★ ★ |

| Physical activity benefit | Surety rating |
|---|---|
| **Nutrition and diet quality** | |
| Improvement in diet quality | ★ ★ |
| Increase in total energy intake | ★ ★ ★ |
| **Sleep** | |
| Improvement in sleep quality | ★ ★ ★ |
| **Weight management** | |
| Prevention of weight gain | ★ ★ ★ ★ |
| Treatment of obesity | ★ ★ |
| Maintenance of weight loss | ★ ★ ★ |
| **Psychological well-being** | |
| Elevation in mood | ★ ★ ★ ★ |
| Buffering of effects of mental stress | ★ ★ ★ |
| Alleviation/prevention of depression | ★ ★ ★ ★ |
| Anxiety reduction | ★ ★ ★ ★ |
| Improvement in self-esteem | ★ ★ ★ ★ |
| **Children and youth** | |
| Prevention of obesity | ★ ★ ★ |
| Control of disease risk factors | ★ ★ ★ |
| Reduction of unhealthy habits | ★ ★ |
| Improved odds of adult activity | ★ ★ |
| **Special issues for women** | |
| Improved total body fitness | ★ ★ ★ ★ |
| Improved fitness while pregnant | ★ ★ ★ ★ |
| Improved birthing experience | ★ ★ |
| Improved health of fetus | ★ ★ |
| Improved health during menopause | ★ ★ ★ |
| **Elderly and the aging process** | |
| Improvement in physical fitness | ★ ★ ★ ★ |
| Countering of loss in heart/lung fitness | ★ ★ |
| Countering of loss of muscle | ★ ★ ★ |
| Countering of gain in fat | ★ ★ ★ |
| Improvement in life expectancy | ★ ★ ★ ★ |
| Improvement in life quality | ★ ★ ★ ★ |

[1] Table is based on a total physical fitness program that includes physical activity designed to improve both aerobic and musculoskeletal fitness.

★ ★ ★ ★ Strong consensus, with little or no conflicting data.

★ ★ ★ Most data are supportive, but more research is needed for clarification.

★ ★ Some data are supportive, but much more research is needed.

★ Little or no data support.

Notice from table 22.1 that the highest "surety ratings" support the idea that regular physical activity improves health in the following ways:

- Reduces the risk of dying prematurely (i.e., improves life expectancy).
- Reduces the risk of dying from heart disease.
- Reduces the risk of developing diabetes.
- Helps prevent and treat high blood pressure.
- Reduces the risk of developing colon cancer.
- Reduces feelings of depression and anxiety while improving mood state and self-esteem.
- Helps control body weight.
- Helps build and maintain healthy bones and muscles and improve heart and lung fitness.
- Improves the life quality of older adults, patients with disease, and people of all ages.

In light of all these health benefits, it is quite amazing that 6 in 10 Americans do not achieve the recommended amount of regular physical activity. Time is the greatest barrier to physical activity, according to most surveys. A team of international experts has urged that legislative bodies strive to pass policies that make it easier for people to include physical activity within their daily routines. Among their recommendations are the following:

- Change building codes to require easy-to-find and inviting stairways.
- Require developers and planners to provide more parks and exercise facilities so that access is convenient for all.
- Bar direct automobile access to the core of cities and provide attractive footpaths, walking and jogging trails, and cycling paths that would encourage people to transport themselves from one place to another by their own power.
- Require physical activity programs that are readily available to all in schools, work sites, community centers, and parks.
- Pass tax legislation that would encourage products and services that promote physical activity.

People are admonished to develop more of an exercise mentality through which they seek to facilitate physical activity instead of raising

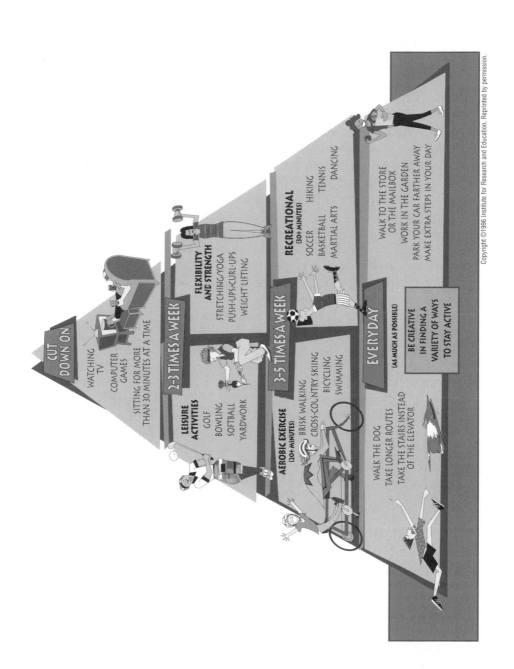

**CUT DOWN ON**
WATCHING TV
COMPUTER GAMES
SITTING FOR MORE THAN 30 MINUTES AT A TIME

**2-3 TIMES A WEEK**

**FLEXIBILITY AND STRENGTH**
STRETCHING/YOGA
PUSH-UPS/CURL-UPS
WEIGHT LIFTING

**LEISURE ACTIVITIES**
GOLF
BOWLING
SOFTBALL
YARDWORK

**RECREATIONAL**
(30+ MINUTES)
SOCCER      HIKING
BASKETBALL      TENNIS
MARTIAL ARTS      DANCING

**3-5 TIMES A WEEK**

**AEROBIC EXERCISE**
(20+ MINUTES)
BRISK WALKING
CROSS-COUNTRY SKIING
BICYCLING
SWIMMING

**EVERYDAY**
(AS MUCH AS POSSIBLE)

**BE CREATIVE IN FINDING A VARIETY OF WAYS TO STAY ACTIVE**

WALK TO THE STORE OR THE MAILBOX
WORK IN THE GARDEN
PARK YOUR CAR FARTHER AWAY
MAKE EXTRA STEPS IN YOUR DAY

WALK THE DOG
TAKE LONGER ROUTES
TAKE THE STAIRS INSTEAD OF THE ELEVATOR

barriers to excuse inactivity. To ensure long-term success, it is necessary to weave physical activity within the daily routine and to be creative in finding a variety of ways to stay active. The Institute for Research and Education HealthSystem Minnesota has produced the "Activity Pyramid" (see figure 22.2), which is an easy-to-follow guide to help people be more physically active. It is based on the successful "Food Pyramid" that has helped people make better food choices.

In 1979, *Healthy People,* a landmark report from the Surgeon General, was published, marking the dawn of a new era in which health promotion and disease prevention became leading priorities among national and state public health leaders. In this report it was noted that "the linked concepts of disease prevention and health promotion are certainly not novel . . . in classical Greece, the followers of the gods of medicine associated the healing arts not only with the god Aesculapius but with his two daughters, Panacea and Hygeia. While Panacea was involved with medication of the sick, her sister Hygeia was concerned with living wisely and preserving health."

This book has attempted to provide you with every reason for finding time to exercise in order that you might preserve your health. Dr. Paul Dudley White, physician to President Eisenhower, believed that "a five-mile walk will do more good for an unhappy but otherwise healthy adult than all the medicine and psychology in the world." Hippocrates had also argued that walking is the best medicine, while Thomas Jefferson upheld the idea that "the sovereign invigorator of the body is exercise, and of all exercises, walking is the best." Modern-day men and women have nearly lost the use of their legs, and the challenge laid before you in this book is to find the health and joy that come in using them.

> Now shall I walk
> or shall I ride?
> "Ride," Pleasure said;
> "Walk," Joy replied.

# REFERENCES

Blair, S.N., Booth, M., Gyarfas, I., et al. (1996). Development of public policy and physical activity initiatives internationally. *Sports Medicine, 21,* 157-163.

Davison, R.C.R., & Grant, S. (1993). Is walking sufficient exercise for health? *Sports Medicine, 16,* 369-373.

Elrick, H. (1996). Exercise is medicine. *The Physician and Sportsmedicine, 24* (2), 72-78.

Fentem, P.H. (1994). Benefits of exercise in health and disease. *British Medical Journal, 308*, 1291-1295.

Haskell, W.L. (1994). Health consequences of physical activity: Understanding and challenges regarding dose-response. *Medicine and Science in Sports and Exercise, 26*, 649-660.

King, A.C. (1994). Community and public health approaches to the promotion of physical activity. *Medicine and Science in Sports and Exercise, 26*, 1405-1412.

Lee, I-M., & Paffenbarger, R.S. (1996). Do physical activity and physical fitness avert premature mortality? *Exercise and Sports Science Reviews, 24*, 135-169.

NIH Consensus Development Panel on Physical Activity and Cardiovascular Health. (1996). Physical activity and cardiovascular health. *Journal of the American Medical Association, 276*, 241-246.

Paffenbarger, R.S., & Lee, I-M. (1996). Physical activity and fitness for health and longevity. *Research Quarterly for Exercise and Sport, 67* (Suppl.), 11-28.

Pate, R.R., Pratt, M., Blair, S.N., et al. (1995). Physical activity and public health: A recommendation from the Centers for Disease Control and Prevention and the American College of Sports Medicine. *Journal of the American Medical Association, 273*, 402-407.

Powell, K.E., & Blair, S.N. (1994). The public health burdens of sedentary living habits: Theoretical but realistic estimates. *Medicine and Science in Sports and Exercise, 26*, 851-856.

U.S. Department of Health and Human Services. (1996). *Physical activity and health: A report of the Surgeon General.* Atlanta: U.S. Department of Health and Human Services, Centers for Disease Control and Prevention, National Center for Chronic Disease Prevention and Health Promotion.

# INDEX

# ABOUT THE AUTHOR

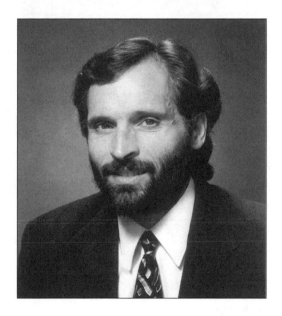

David C. Nieman, DrPH, FACSM, has been a professor of health and exercise science for more than 25 years. He currently teaches at Appalachian State University in Boone, North Carolina. Not only is he the author of several books, including *Fitness and Sports Medicine: A Health-Related Approach*, *Nutritional Assessment*, and *Fitness and Your Health*, but he has written more than 200 articles that have appeared in such publications as *Women's Sports and Fitness*, *ACE Fitness Matters*, and *Vibrant Life*. He is also on the editorial boards of the *International Journal of Sport Nutrition*, *Sports Medicine*, *Training and Rehabilitation*, and *Exercise Immunology Annual*.

Nieman received a doctorate in public health from Loma Linda University in California in 1984. In addition to being a Fellow of the American College of Sports Medicine, he is certified as a Health/Fitness Instructor by that organization. He is also a member of the American Public Health Association and the American Physiological Society.

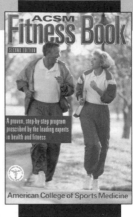
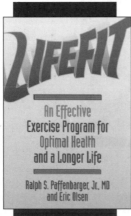
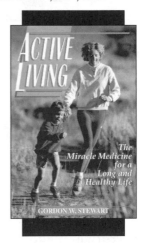